Behind Closed Doors

Outspoken
Series Editor: Neda Tehrani

Platforming underrepresented voices; intervening in important political issues; revealing powerful histories and giving voice to our experiences; Outspoken is a series unlike any other. Unravelling debates on sex education, masculinity, feminism, mental health, and class and inequality, Outspoken has the answers to the questions you're asking. These are books that dissent.

Also available:

Mask Off
Masculinity Redefined
JJ Bola

Feminism, Interrupted
Disrupting Power
Lola Olufemi

Split
Class Divides Uncovered
Ben Tippet

Behind Closed Doors

Sex Education Transformed

Natalie Fiennes

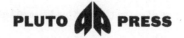

First published 2019 by Pluto Press
345 Archway Road, London N6 5AA

www.plutobooks.com

Copyright © Natalie Fiennes 2019

The right of Natalie Fiennes to be identified as the author of this
work has been asserted by her in accordance with the Copyright,
Designs and Patents Act 1988.

British Library Cataloguing in Publication Data
A catalogue record for this book is available from the British Library

ISBN   978 0 7453 3873 6   Paperback
ISBN   978 1 7868 0499 0   PDF eBook
ISBN   978 1 7868 0501 0   Kindle eBook
ISBN   978 1 7868 0500 3   EPUB eBook

This book is printed on paper suitable for recycling and made
from fully managed and sustained forest sources. Logging, pulping
and manufacturing processes are expected to conform to the
environmental standards of the country of origin.

Typeset by Stanford DTP Services, Northampton, England

Simultaneously printed in the United Kingdom and United States of
America

Contents

Acknowledgements

To all the extraordinary young people I spoke to writing this book: your inspiration kept me going. To my friends and my editor: Neda, the Fiennes family, Ben, Lydia, Laetitia, Otti, Hannah, Sam, Harriet, Emma, Joanna, Naomi, Vida, Lily and Elly. And to the many more who held my hand along the way.

Introduction

She may be a bag of trouble: A short history of sex education

I had my first sex education class when I was eleven. We piled into the classroom and sat down in rows facing a tiny blank screen. We were mostly naive and almost entirely bored. When the teacher came in she explained that we were about to watch a video of a woman giving birth. She reassured us that yes, we might feel a bit queasy, but not to worry because it was all very natural and normal and besides, this is how we all came into the world. She pressed play. Within seconds one of the boys fainted. He slid off his stool and crumpled, whimpering, into a mound of oversized blazer on the floor. It was terrifying – the perfect contraceptive.

The next (and final) instalment took place when I was 13. In this session, the school's agonised vicar muttered under his breath about teen pregnancies, the horrors of AIDS and the very precise symptoms of gonorrhoea. After an initial preamble, he opened up the ominous black briefcase he had brought along with him. Lo and behold, it contained – behind a very thick pane of glass – an intriguing selection of small plastic bags, white powders, pill packets and green herbs. He awkwardly gestured towards

1

the morning after pill, a bag of cocaine, a diaphragm and a bag of weed. The briefcase was slammed shut and we were dismissed.

As I would discover researching for this book, most young people in the UK might have some semblance of a sex education at school, but school was not where they learned about sex. Some might have been taught by religious leaders or family members, but the overwhelming majority were left to fend for themselves, asking sly questions to friends and older siblings, learning by mistake, looking this-and-that up online, and always, always finding an excuse to scuttle away when the topic was breached by parents. Despite the torments, I presumed that things were better than they had been in the past. Surely the awkwardness of my school's vicar was preferable to those vicars of the past – railing about sin, blindness and the fiery pits of eternal damnation.

Sex education has changed wildly throughout time and continues to vary around the world today. This should come as no surprise. The way that sex education comes to be taught – or indeed not taught – depends on some pretty central questions. Take the very idea of a young person. What does it mean to be young? Is it to be innocent? Irrational? Reckless? And what even is the role of education? Is it something that should be left to parents? Maybe it's corrupting to teach children about 'adult' things. And what about sex? What is normal sex? Or good sex? Is it for procreation? For spiritual and religious ends? But what about non-heterosexual sex? And what about gender? Or marriage?

An American school board member wrote in 1986, 'There's an old saying that "there are only two things for certain in this world; death and taxes," a third certainly might be added: disagreement about sex education.'[1] Sex is extremely personal, arguably the

---

1   Sherry Martschink, 'Somewhere, Somehow, Children Must Get an Education in Sex,' *News and Courier* (Charleston, South Carolina, 2 August 1986); 'South Carolina Sex Education Clippings folder,' box 250, *James T. Sears Papers* (Duke University, Durham, North Carolina).

highest form of intimacy of all, but it is also connected to a complicated web of forces outside of the self. From culture, religion, class, race, gender, all the way to the randomness of which constituency you grow up in and how much funding your school receives, sex is political.

The seeds of sex ed

Formal sex education as we know it now might not have been around for long, but sex education has always existed. Before printing presses and even before classrooms were introduced, knowledge was transferred between generations by word of mouth: through fables, myth and stories.

Thousands of years ago in parts of what we now call India, learning about healthy relationships was considered an essential part of moving into adulthood. The Sanskrit *Kamasutra*, written around 400BC, is famed for its practical advice for newly-weds, but it also taught that erotic love is only one part of a spiritually rich and fulfilling adult life.[2] One thousand years later, this approach prevailed in Hindu communities. Take, for instance, the Khajuraho Temple Complex in Northern India, built around 1,000 years ago for both Hindus and Jains. The temple is covered from floor to ceiling with hundreds upon hundreds of erotic carvings; of people on their own, in pairs, in groups and even with animals. The temple was a place of worship, but also a space for learning.

Parts of India were so sexually liberal that the swinging sixties pale in comparison. So, what happened? Around the time that Khajuraho was built, the other side of the world was undergoing a revolution in thought. In spite of intense and violent persecution, a new religion had broken from Judaism and was spreading throughout Europe. Through the life of Jesus, it spoke of human

---

2 Mallanaga Vatsyayana, *Kamasutra* (Oxford: Oxford University Press, 2009).

suffering, of everlasting life, forgiveness and the spiritual importance of marriage.

When the Portuguese set off in search of riches and adventure, landing on the shores of West Africa in 1498, they ensured that the Christian revolution would be a global revolution. From the 1500s to the 1960s, other European powers followed their lead and became the largest empire in history. Britain alone has invaded almost 90 per cent of countries around the world.[3]

Europeans obviously do not have a monopoly on violence. Japan and Turkey both had their own brutal empires and before the invasion of the East India Company in India, the Mughals were enormously repressive, killing tens of thousands of people in the quest for land. The later Moguls, in particular, also imposed extremely conservative values on their population, well before the British arrived. However, in the words of British rapper and author Akala, 'the idea of race and white supremacy pioneered in eighteenth-century Europe, combined with newly formed nation states and industrial technology, took the human capacity for and practice of barbarity to levels rarely if ever before seen in history.'[4] This barbarity included imposing a very particular and narrow understanding of human nature, and specifically in relation to this book, human sexuality.

Colonial expansion wasn't just a way to collect wealth and build an empire: it was also about changing minds. In the words of Aimé Césaire, the Martinique poet and politician, it was a 'campaign to civilise barbarism', built upon the idea of the 'overall superiority of Western civilisation over exotic civilisations'.[5] Take a look at

---

3 Stuart Laycock, *All the Countries We've Ever Invaded: And the Few We Never Got Round To* (Stroud: The History Press, 2012).

4 Akala, *Natives: Race and Class in the Ruins of Empire* (London: Two Roads Books, 2018).

5 Aimé Césaire, 'Discourse on Colonialism,' translated by Joan Pinkham (New York and London: Monthly Review Press, 1972).

this quote from the travel diary of a German foot soldier from the fourteenth century:

> In the land of Indian there are men with dog's heads who talk by barking [and] . . . feed by catching birds . . . Others again have only one eye in the forehead [. . .] Close to Paradise on the River Ganges who eat nothing. For they absorb liquid nourishment through a straw and live on the juice of flowers . . . Many have such large under lips that they can cover their whole faces with them.[6]

These travellers' tales became legend. If you were a fourteenth century Englishman, how else would you come to learn about other cultures around world? While there certainly were many racist and fantastical accounts, like the one above, not all explorers were so blatantly derogatory. In fact, many were consumed by awe.

When the British explorer Captain Cook arrived in Tahiti in 1769, he wrote back home with descriptions of what can only be described as a sexual paradise. He spoke of women, more beautiful and more willing than anyone you'd meet on the dreary British Isles.[7] The Tahitian women are depicted just like fruit: readily available, exotic and for the enjoyment of European globetrotters. Just because the representation is seemingly positive, can we say it's any less objectifying? As we will see throughout the book, these radicalised stereotypes of the past still haunt us today.[8]

Cook might have marvelled at what he saw as a kind of sexual innocence, untainted by Christian shame, but many in the Church had a different perspective. Christian missionaries worked closely

---

6   E. Newby, *The Mitchell Beazley World Atlas of Exploration* (London: Mitchell Beazley, 1975), 17.

7   Peter Moore, *Endeavour: The Ship and the Attitude that Changed the World* (London: Chatto & Windus, 2018).

8   Stuart Hall and Bram Gieben, *Formations of Modernity* (Cambridge: Polity Press, 1992).

with colonial powers to spread the word of God. Tens of thousands of churches were built around the world where millions of people were given free food, clean water and access to safe medical care. Nonetheless, at the heart of this mission was a fundamental belief in the superiority of Western thought over other traditions, and that the use of violence and force to maintain that domination was permissible. Within the Church's teachings were strict ideas about sex and marriage, and in an unprecedented move, the Church introduced the first global sex education in human history.

Enter the Victorians

As the nineteenth century rolled in, the Industrial Revolution saw that Western countries went through astronomical upheavals. Victorians knew they were living through tumultuous times: 'We who lived before railways were made belong to another world. It was only yesterday, but what a gulf between now and then!' wrote the novelist William Thackeray in 1860, 'we who survive out of the ancient world are like Father Noah and his family out of the ark.'[9] With such great technological upheaval, and hundreds of thousands travelling away from small villages towards growing urban hubs, we can identify similarities between the Victorian era and the present day. Much like today, social values were also in flux.

Victorians tend to be remembered as fuddy-duddy, sexually repressed antiques, but as many historians will tell you, this doesn't quite hold up. Not only was it the birth of smutty pornography, but there was just as much pleasure seeking in 1860 as you'd find a hundred years later. The population was booming, STI rates were through the roof and poverty was pushing increasing numbers of women to sex work.[10] Major changes to sexuality came from

9   William M. Thackeray, 'De Juventute,' *Roundabout Papers and Other Works* (New York: Simon and Schuster, 2014).

10   Matthew Sweet, *Inventing the Victorians* (London: Faber and Faber, 2002).

above. The fear that overpopulation would lead to the collapse of society was held as fact and the institutions of power – the law, the Church, the medical establishment – sharpened their focus on sex. It became a matter for public concern, and nowhere more so than in the new so-called science of 'sexology'.

Sexologists set out to define the true nature of human sexuality, but their conclusions more or less repeated the same values already advocated by society: that heterosexuality is the norm, that gender is binary, that women are passive and men are active, and masturbation is dangerous. As we will explore throughout the book, these values still dominate.

'She may look clean . . . but'

It wasn't until World War One that Western governments created the first sex education programmes. Take a read of this British soldier's memoir of the war:

> There were well over a hundred and fifty men waiting for opening time, singing Mademoiselle from Armentiéres and other lusty songs. Right on the dot of 6 PM a red lamp over the doorway of the brothel was switched on. A roar went up from the troops, accompanied by a forward lunge towards the entrance . . .[11]

In the trenches, brothels displayed blue lamps for officers and red for other ranks. The red lamps would draw thrumming crowds of men, but this was especially true before a major offensive, where those soldiers who believed it was their last night alive would choose not to spend it alone. Twenty-four hours before the 1915 Battle of Loos (where 59,247 British soldiers lost their lives) one

11   George Coppard, *With a Machine Gun to Cambrai: The Tale of a Young Tommy in Kitchener's Army 1914–1918* (London: H.M.S.O, 1969), 56

soldier recalls seeing 'three hundred men in a queue, all waiting their turns to go in the Red Lamp [. . .] I suppose that subconsciously we wanted as much of life as we could get while we still had life.'[12] Claiming the lives of over 16 million soldiers, World War I was deadly, but it also opened the door to an explosion of sexually transmitted diseases, or venereal diseases (VD) as they were called then. The figures are astonishing: in 1916 one in five of every British troop admitted to hospital in France and Belgium was due to an STI.[13] That also takes into consideration trench foot and all other kinds of injuries resulting from conflict.

Frisky soldiers became a great embarrassment to allied governments so they took action. Condoms were handed out to soldiers for free and large chunks of money were allocated to sex education. When fresh British soldiers set off for the trenches they were each given a letter from the Secretary of State for War, Lord Kitchener reading thus: 'in this new experience you may find temptations both in wine and women. You must entirely resist both.' In the words of one solider, Private Frank Richards: 'They may as well have not been issued for all the notice we took of them.'

American soldiers were also given reading material on the front. One pamphlet, called *When You Go Home – Take This Book With You*, starts with this: 'You have won the war against autocracy. The fight against venereal diseases – as base a hypocrite, as foul a murderer as any Hun [German] – has only just begun!'[14] It doesn't stop there. The leaflet concludes that: 'The only sure way to keep from getting clap [gonorrhoea] and syphilis is to keep away from prostitutes or other loose women . . . It is not necessary to go with women to keep well. All athletes know this. The fact that famous boxers and

---

12   www.bbc.co.uk/news/uk-england-25762151 (last accessed 03/2019).
13   www.bbc.co.uk/news/uk-england-25762151 (last accessed 20/11/2018).
14   https://archive.org/details/WhenYouGoHome.

wrestlers keep away from women while in training proves that a man is even stronger when he does not go with them'.[15]

As these words show, women were blamed for the rise in STIs. In the UK, the trope of the whorish, dirty, disease-infected woman reared its ugly head when posters were plastered over the walls of the country saying things like 'She May be a Bag of Trouble' and 'She May Look Clean – BUT . . . pick-ups, "good time" girls, prostitutes SPREAD SYPHILIS AND GONORRHOEA'. The British government took prompt action against women. In 1916, the UK made it illegal for sex workers to approach men in uniform. In 1918, further regulation gave power to the police to medically examine any woman they suspected to be a prostitute. Given that so many men were killed at war, plunging their wives and family back home into poverty, large numbers of women relied on sex work as a survival mechanism. In practice the policy meant that poor women – or people the police wanted to harass – were pulled off the streets and forcibly given a medical examination. This misogynist legislation, which was so obviously designed to protect men and denigrate women, led to such fierce protests from the suffragette movement that it was eventually revoked.[16]

Missionary presses

The last 100 years have seen sex education programmes becoming the norm. However, in the 1920s, they did not always spring from the best intentions.

Much like in India, many pre- and early colonial indigenous communities in South Africa viewed sex education as an integral part of young people's entrance into the world. With the arrival

---

15   https://archive.org/details/WhenYouGoHome.
16   S. Buckley, 'The failure to resolve the problem of venereal disease among the troops in Britain during World War I,' in B. Bond et al. (eds.), *War and Society: A Yearbook of Military History*, vol. 2 (New York: Holmes and Meier, 1977), 65–85.

of the Dutch and then the British, this changed. In deeply racist 1920s South African society, white and black inter-racial relationships were viewed as a perversion of the highest degree, and white children from settler communities were given the strictest of instructions to refrain from any kind of mixing. With this intention in mind, the 1920s saw a number of Christian printing presses set up, called – without a whiff of irony – 'missionary presses'. One of the most popular educational pamphlets distributed was called *Facts about Ourselves for Growing Boys and Girls* and, unusually for its time, it actually encouraged the young white readership to have lots of sex. 'It is your duty' the author writes, 'to help your race to progress'.[17]

Back in 1920s London, one in ten people in the capital had syphilis and a new government sex education department – who happened to be sharing an office with the Eugenics team – had produced the UK's first sex ed pamphlets for school children.[18] Within 20 years, Britain was at war again and facing the same problems as they did during World War One. There were concerns about 'lowering moral standards inevitable in war-time', 'the temptation to seize the pleasure of the moment without regard for the future' and an 'unfortunate fatalism'.[19,20]

During the latter part of the twentieth century, the number of young people around the world going to school exploded. By 1985, 90 per cent of the world's children had spent at least some part of

---

17   Sarah Emily Duff, 'Let's talk about sex education: race and shame in South Africa,' https://theconversation.com/lets-talk-about-sex-education-race-and-shame-in-south-africa-41390 (last accessed 10/09/2018).

18   Jonathan Zimmerman, *Too Hot to Handle* (Oxford: Princeton University Press, 2015).

19   J. Ewing, 'Sex education in schools,' *Health Education Journal* 2, no. 1 (1944): 11–18.

20   M. H. Bennett, 'Sex beliefs and behaviour,' *Health Education Journal* 3, no. 2 (1945): 84–7.

their lives at school.[21] This rise coincided with a number of legal changes in the West throughout the 1960s. In the UK, the contraceptive pill was legalised; homosexuality decriminalised; abortion legalised and the first challenges by trans people addressing gender identity were brought to the courts. By 1970, condoms were free on the NHS by request, regardless of marital status or age.

These massive changes opened up questions about how to support, educate and control the sexuality of future generations of young people. It is common for there to be unease talking about childhood sexuality, and for many important reasons. However, advocates for sex education see it as essential to empower young people with the age-appropriate facts. In spite of the general trajectory towards global sex education teaching, there have always been critics who worry about corrupting 'innocent minds'. This was evident in the case of Sweden, which in 1959 became the first country in the world to have compulsory sex ed classes. However, there were many in Sweden who feared these changes, with some saying that sex education in schools might 'awaken the sleeping bear'. Swedish critics were not alone. It was also during this period that Japanese opponents suggested that sex education would 'wake a sleeping child'. In Vietnam critics said that it was like 'showing the way to the deer' and in Thailand that it was like 'showing nuts to the squirrel'.[22]

In the end it was panic and hasty measures that pushed the UK government into implementing the national sex education programs that young people, such as myself, had in our childhood. It was the devastation caused by the 1980s AIDS epidemic which swept like wildfire through the world that sent the nation into

---

21 John W. Meyer et al., 'The World's Educational Revolution, 1950–1970,' *Sociology of Education* 50, no. 4 (1977): 244; John W. Meyer, Francisco O. Ramirez, and Yasemin Nuhoglu Soysal, 'World Expansion of Mass Education, 1870–1980,' *Sociology of Education* 65, no. 2 (1992): 128.

22 Jonathan Zimmerman, *Too Hot to Handle* (Oxford: Princeton University Press, 2015).

panic about deadly sexually transmitted diseases and – fired by the British press – creeping homosexuality and moral attack to family values. The AIDS crisis forced the UK government to implement sex education programmes based on public education, safe sex practices and disease prevention. International institutions like the UN and the World Health Organisation (WHO) put pressure on countries in the Global South to follow suit.

The 1990s saw another moral panic, but this time around it was teen pregnancies. A vicious characterisation of a working-class single mother, dependent on welfare benefits emerged. Not unlike attitudes towards gay men in the 1980s, this characterisation was looming in the background when the Conservative government introduced the 1993 Education Act, which stated that all state schools had to provide some sort of sex education 'in such a manner as to encourage young people to have regard to moral considerations and the value of family life'. Parents had to consent to these classes, and there was always an option to pull their children out.

Where are we now?

We land in the present. On 1 March 2017, the UK government ruled that come September 2020, sex and relationship education will be compulsory in the UK. This is a historic moment in education. But question marks remain over what it will look like in practice.

As we've seen, sex education programmes tend to reflect the politics of the time. The 1980s saw a huge push from the UK government towards universal comprehensive sex ed, but it occurred in the midst of a largely homophobic society. It was during this period that then Prime Minister Margaret Thatcher passed a law which explicitly forbade the 'promotion of homosexuality' by local councils, preventing schools from teaching about any kind of sexuality that wasn't strictly heterosexual, and promoting so-called 'family values'. This law was only overturned by Labour in 2003.

In this book, I've spoken to people from around the country about what kind of sex education they would like. I've drawn on histories and testimonies, on politics and on culture to try and bring the conversation to where we, as young people, want it to be. Because despite thousands of years to-ing and fro-ing, all research done that actually asks young people what they want from sex education says the same thing: that there should be one, that it should be honest, age appropriate, taught without embarrassment and that it should be relevant.

Chapter 1

Sex: 'I am fast'

Gender equality does not trouble Chacma baboons. Originating from Namibia, they are some of the largest and most boisterous monkeys in the world. A fully grown male weighs almost double that of the female, and he relishes his position at the top of the pack: hoarding the best food, lording over his turf and even fighting with leopards to maintain his position. In matters of the heart, he's just as machismo. He picks his choice female in the weeks leading up to her ovulation, attacking her, chasing her, and withholding food until she succumbs. Violence against the females is not only common, but central to the most successful seductions; the more aggressive the male the more likely the female is to mate with him.

Generations of people have looked to the animal world to draw conclusions about the behaviour of humans. Baboons are indeed our close cousins. We share many traits: our blood clots in a similar way, both species have 'cumulative culture' – the incredible ability to pass knowledge down through generations – and we even use some of the same vowels that are essential for speech. But what can we learn from baboons about our own sex and gender? It has been claimed that the 'natural' and rigid gendered hierarchies of baboons tells us something about our own natural state, placing a limit on feminist demands for gender equality and fluidity.

Yet, even if we accept the idea that our original sexual state of nature was/is hierarchical and rigidly defined – a premise we will interrogate later – the argument above falls prey to what philosophers have long called 'the genetic fallacy'. The fallacy arises from giving credit to the origin of something, even when that origin is no longer relevant. You can see the fallacy clearly in the following example. Chemistry arose from the study of Alchemy, a superstitious discipline that aimed to turn lead into gold. But does this mean that Chemistry is unscientific because Alchemy is unscientific? Clearly it does not. Likewise, any argument about gender and sex that relies solely on an origin story, rather than acknowledging how human behaviour adapts and changes with the times, falls prey to the fallacy.

The big, screaming problem with the comparison to the non-human animal world is that we are not baboons. Neither are we ants nor dogs. Comparisons between humans and other animals tends to be both superficial and selective. So what can we say about sex, biology and human character?

Growing up

Rather than going back to our baboon-ancestral state of nature to learn about our biology, let's start with a place we have all actually been: our very first days in the womb. For the first six to seven weeks of life humans appear sexless. Floating around in the womb, all foetuses appear to have identical genitalia until around eight weeks, when a surge of growth hormones kicks in and the blueprint of DNA makes the building blocks of our body. It's at this point that we develop sexual and reproductive organs. For the majority of us they will form male and female body organs, but for around 1.7 per cent of the population – 1.3 million in the UK – they will be born intersex, which as the name suggests, means being born with reproductive or sexual anatomies that don't fit typical definitions of male or female. There are an estimated 30 different ways of being intersex, demonstrating quite how varied human gender actually is.[1] And in spite of such great variety, after birth the first question asked is almost always: is it a boy or a girl?

Like all other living species and creatures on earth, homo sapiens have been separated into two distinct biological categories: male and female. From a medical perspective, someone's sex is determined by five key features – chromosomes, hormones, genitals, secondary sex characteristics (physical features that appear during puberty like breasts, facial hair and Adam's apples) and gonads (ovaries or testes) – but in practice most babies are ascribed a sex based on the appearance of their genitalia.

Gender, on the other hand, is another story. Gender refers to all the social and cultural baggage that we put onto the sexes. It includes the range of behaviours and attributes we commonly associate with male-ness and female-ness, but also our own identity and how we view ourselves (see Chapters 3 and 4). Nonetheless, sex and gender tend to be treated as one and the same thing. Whenever you're required to fill out personal data, there tends to be just two options of 'male' and 'female' (although today Facebook have seventy-one genders and counting, and increasingly other places provide more than two options). Even though the passport register might ask you what your gender is, what they're really asking about is your sex. You would probably be faced with a blank and quite probably hostile look if you told the person processing your debit card application: 'well, I have a penis and often I feel male. Other days I feel both man and women, and sometimes neither!'

Whereas we are ascribed a sex at birth, our gender identity is formed years later. By the ripe age of three most children will prefer activities that are typically associated with their sex and by the age of four or five most children will have a strong sense of their gender. The nature-nurture debate still rages as to what

---

1   Alice Dreger, '"Ambiguous Sex"– or Ambivalent Medicine?' *The Hastings Center Report* (May/Jun 1998) 28, no. 3, 24–35; Fausto-Sterling, Anne, *Sexing The Body: Gender Politics and the Construction of Sexuality* (Basic Books, 2000).

causes this. For some people, they see this as an inescapable, essential path chosen for us by biology and genes. Because these developments take place so early, gender can *appear* very natural. When the gender scholar Michael Kimmel became a father, for instance, he reported that an old friend probed him with glee, Ha! 'Now you'll see it's all biological!'[2] And yet, many others point to the absolute power of repetition, absorption and imitation in these early years, shaping and forming how children are brought into society. But more of that later.

Between the ages of eight and fourteen puberty typically kicks in – it can feel intense because it is intense. Enormous physical changes occur within the body. People gain weight in places that make them feel disproportioned. Hair grows. Sweat starts to smell. Acne appears. Voice changes. Breasts develop. Menstruation begins. Hair grows in previously hairless places. And these are just the physical changes. Pubescent hormones also have a huge impact on the mind during puberty. It's very common for teenagers to feel aggressive, depersonalised, depressed and to experience extreme mood swings. By the end of puberty – which can be well into the twenties for many – the human body and mind has entered adulthood. From breasts, to Adam's apples to facial hair, it's these 'secondary sex' characteristics many develop during puberty that signal to the outside what our sex is.

'I just want to run naturally'

South African Caster Semenya is one of the fastest runners in history. During her first senior competition in the 2009 World Championship in Berlin, she won the 800m race by nearly 2.5 seconds, cruising effortlessly past her competitors. Caster is breathtakingly athletic, she has a strong jawline and her voice is low, or as Caster's father, Jacob, has put it: 'if you speak to her

---

2   Kimmel, 2004, p. vii.

on the telephone, you might mistake her for a man'.[3] As soon as she broke the record people started talking about her. Members of the pubic wrote into the International Association of Athletics Federations (IAAF), the athletics governing body, with complaints and just before she was due to accept her gold medal in Berlin, a reporter broke the story that Semenya's sex was indeed ambiguous and that she had been required to undergo a gender-verification test before the race. The IAAF confirmed the rumour and many of her indignant competitors joined the conversation: 'Just look at her' Mariya Savinova, of Russia, who finished fifth, said.

It was Rupert Murdoch's paper, Australia's *Daily Telegraph,* that leaked the results of Caster's test. It showed she has a hormonal condition known as hyperandrogenism, meaning that her testosterone levels are far higher than average level for females. After the IAAF considered her case, Caster was withdrawn from all international competitions and it wasn't until legal action, and a huge international campaign, that in July 2010 the IAAF cleared her to return to competition. She has since become the first person in history to win all three of the 400m, 800m and 1500m titles – and at the time of writing, she's the reigning world and Olympic 800m champion. Yet there is no respite. The most recent official line is that Caster – and other intersex athletes – have to reduce their testosterone levels to an 'acceptable' level before they can participate.[4] Her struggle continues.

When she returned home, Caster was treated as a hero. In a country that's suffered deep trauma from classifying humans based on biological difference, sports have played an important role in building solidarity across class and race lines. Nelson Mandela himself said that sports are 'more powerful than governments in breaking down racial barriers' and that 'sport has the power to change the world. It has the power to inspire, the power to unite

---

3   www.newyorker.com/magazine/2009/11/30/eitheror Accessed January 2019.
4   www.iaaf.org/news/press-release/eligibility-regulations-for-female-classifica.

people that little else has.' It's ironic then that discrimination has made its way to the heart of South African sporting politics.

The IAAF were forced to answer a question that no-one in history has ever been able to answer: what is the true difference between men and women? Their conclusion was hormones, that high levels of testosterone give female athletes an unfair advantage over their competitors, and that in order to be still considered a female, they need to artificially reduce testosterone levels. It's certainly true that many athletes use testosterone in doping to help build muscle mass and red-blood-production. However, a recent review by two Harvard endocrinologists concluded that it is still 'unclear' whether naturally high testosterone in women, including intersex women, 'confers any competitive advantage' at all.[5] Further still, a number of researchers have come forward to say that the findings of the IAAF are severely flawed and that they should not have used these conclusions to penalise Semenya at all.[6]

Even if we say that testosterone does help with performance, surely having a natural physical advantage over competitors is the point of sports. In the case of Caster, this happens to be hormone levels, but is there ever such a thing as fair game in sports? Isn't athletic achievement always about a combination of natural ability and training?

A conversation that would usually be seen as crude and invasive – Caster's genitalia – has been thrashed out and held to scrutiny by the world. Jennifer Doyle, Professor at the University of California, points out 'no other extraordinary athlete had been singled out with such determination for this form of exile or medical intervention.'[7] It's led the ANC, the ruling party of South Africa, to accuse the IAAF of 'blatant racism'.

5   www.ncbi.nlm.nih.gov/pubmed/28711608.
6   http://bjsm.bmj.com/content/early/2018/02/22/bjsports-2017-098513.info; http://bjsm.bmj.com/content/early/2018/01/18/bjsports-2017-098446.info.
7   https://thesportspectacle.com/2016/08/16/capturing-semenya.

Sometimes being intersex can lead to medical problems, but most intersex people are healthy. Yet there are countless stories from around the world, including the UK, of intersex children who have their sex decided by medical professionals and parents and are operated on in their infant-hood, before they have the capacity to consent. Sometimes the operations and hormonal treatments are necessary for the wellbeing of the child, but more often than not it's due to being misinformed, and more profoundly, the inability of Western societies to negotiate the fact that sex does not work as a binary. The surgeries on intersex people are often irreversible and can lead to physical and emotional scarring: it's the literal application of misguided and stigmatising cultural values around sex onto people's bodies.

Biological fact

Common wisdom today says that there are fundamental, hardwired, physical differences between the sexes, and this physical difference is correlated with differences in behaviour and attributes. This perspective is echoed and reinforced everywhere: there are best-selling books on the topic; countless articles in the press; films that include throw away comments about men being one way and women being another way; toys for girls and boys in separate aisles; and it's not uncommon to hear comments like 'boys will be boys'; 'boys don't cry' or 'girls don't like a sissy'. The idea that the sexes are distinct and essentially different is so entrenched that it tends to be accepted as fact, even within academic communities. In the words of Cambridge University's celebrity psychologist Simon Baron-Cohen (and cousin of Ali G and Borat actor Sasha Baron Cohen) 'the female brain is predominantly hard-wired for empathy. The male brain is predominantly hard-wired for understanding and building systems'.[8]

---

8   Simon Baron-Cohen, *The Essential Difference: Men, Women and the Extreme Male Brain* (London: Penguin, 2003), 1.

Yet, the two claims the argument rests on – (i) there are clear physical differences between the sexes, and (ii) these physical differences are correlated with personal traits – are not a given.

Let's start with the first premise. Can people be clearly categorized into two sexes based on the five characteristics we started this chapter with – chromosomes, hormones, genitals, secondary sex characteristics and gonads (ovaries or testes)? Since most people will never have their chromosomes tested and few people have their hormones checked, the key indicator of sex tends to be secondary sex characteristics – the physical attributes most typically associated with male/female.

All secondary sex characteristics can be changed. People born with a vagina can take testosterone – ending up with a deeper voice and more facial hair. If someone assigned female takes male hormones before puberty, they may actually never experience the development of any secondary sex characteristics. If a woman has her ovaries removed after ovarian cancer, does that make her any less of a woman? Or breasts removed after breast cancer? There is not a medical basis to understanding sex purely in binary terms.

'Testosterone has long featured prominently in explanations of the differences between the sexes, and continues to do so,' eminent philosopher Cordelia Fine argues in *Testosterone Rex*. 'It tends to be enough to say 'Testosterone' to persuade some people that 'boys will be boys''. Fine shows, however, that even though there's no question that hormones affect our bodies, brain and behaviour, there's no evidence that they are more important than other biological and environmental factors. As Fine argues: 'there are no essential male or female characteristics—not even when it comes to risk taking and competitiveness, the traits so often called on to explain why men are more likely to rise to the top.'[9]

---

9 Cordelia Fine, *Testosterone Rex: Myths of Sex, Science and Society* (W.W. Norton & Company, 2017).

In the words of Katrina Karkazis, author of *Fixing Sex: Intersex, Medical Authority, and Lived Experience*: 'To reduce sex to a single trait is to profoundly mischaracterise decades of research into sex biology. The science is clear: there is no single physiological or biological marker that allows for the simple categorisation of people as male or female.'[10] The reality is far more complicated. The fact that the IAAF keep changing their own definitions of who is a 'real woman' and who isn't, should give us some indication about how complicated this question really is.

What the relentless stream of debate around sexual difference really reveals is a drive to find some kind of biological or material basis for something that is fundamentally a social construct: gender inequality. In reality, there is enormous biological difference even within the sexes. One cis-man's experience with their sex will not be identical to another's. Finally, and perhaps most importantly, gender and sex are not the only fault-lines between us. There are many other factors that inform and shape identity, experience and behaviour – whether that's race, class, ability or anything else. Human sexuality and gender identity are tremendously complex yet we have narrow-mindedly categorised sex into two binary camps.

Caster's story shows the real-life consequences of holding these values so dear. There is no such thing as a 'true sex'. It's by understanding why these categories were created in the first place that we can begin to incorporate a much broader, flexible and ultimately accepting definition of what it means to have a sex and gender: one that is founded in human experience, and not – as many might prefer – the mating habits of baboons.

---

10 www.theguardian.com/commentisfree/2019/mar/06/testosterone-biological-sex-sports-bodies.

Chapter 2

Gender identity: Changing rooms

In November 2017, Topshop found itself at the heart of a fierce debate about trans rights. The Manchester branch of Sir Phillip Green's shopping chain had barred artist and activist Travis Alabanza (pronoun they) from entering a women's changing room, despite a new company policy, which said that anyone, regardless of gender, could use either male or female changing rooms.

Later that day, Travis tweeted:

Hey @Topshop just experienced transphobia in your Manchester store. Not letting me use the changing room I decide is shit, sort it out. Gendered changing rooms, effect and put queer and trans shoppers at risk from harassment from other shoppers. It's dated and dangerous.

Travis' tweet promoted a flurry of articles and, as usual, a torrent of abuse. Travis faced death threats, their personal details were leaked, their house was targeted and their neighbours were contacted, 'outing' Travis in the process. Suddenly thrown into the limelight, Travis's identity and life was paraded in front of a public which then dissected, ridiculed and shamed Travis: 'Lmfaoo I see demons when I look at your kind,' was one of the softer comments, which is saying something. Just like Caster Semenya, and the public trials of medieval witches, Travis found themself strung out before the unforgiving court of public opinion.

As this is a particularly explosive and expansive topic, it's important to note that I'm taking a narrow focus, looking at the treatment of trans and gender non-conforming people in the media, and the law. I'll be sticking closely to the accounts and experiences of people who are actually trans or gender-queer – and unpicking some of the most dangerous narratives that society holds about gender non-conformity.

Variety

We know that people who do not identity with the sex they were given at birth have always existed. Yet what many today call 'The Trans Issue' is spoken about as if it is a modern phenomenon. In reality, all of history, religious and cultural traditions, ancient mythology and even fairy tales tell us that there is nothing new about gender fluidity. What's changed is how society treats it.

Whereas most of the world today treats gender non-conforming people with stigma and misunderstanding, this hasn't always been the way. In Ancient Greek mythology, Tiresias, the (male) blind prophet of Apollo, spent seven years as a woman, gaining deep and profound insight into human nature and was given heroic status as a result.

Similarly, in some strands of the Hindu tradition, gender is understood as a weakness. Whereas many of the gods are genderless, humans are afflicted by the limitations of division. Trans, gender non-conforming or intersex people (called 'hijras') have therefore held a particularly special place in Indian tradition for thousands of years, and are revered alongside the gods in holy texts such as the *Mahabharata* and the *Kama Sutra* for transcending gender. Hijra were not just venerated in Hinduism; they also held important spiritual positions in early Mughal courts. It wasn't until the later more conservative Mughals and then the British Invasion of India that they came to be vilified and persecuted. In 1897, the English passed a law that criminalised all Hijras and codified decades of marginalisation and oppression. The law was only undone in 2014.

Changing rooms

On 11 November 2017, days after Travis's tweet, *Times* journalist Janice Turner reported the story under the headline 'Children Sacrificed to Appease Trans Lobby'. In the piece Turner argued that Travis, and other non-binary and trans-feminine people, were a threat to children and should not be allowed to use female changing rooms. However, she claimed, because of the power of trans people and trans allies, this danger had been ignored in what she described as a 'mindless rush to appear right on.'[1]

Her piece entered the swelling number of comment and thought pieces on 'the trans issue'. Greater education and awareness around gender variety can only be a good thing, but very often mainstream discussion boils down to whether trans people are lying about who they are: the 'trans debate' becomes about trans existence. From this perspective, Turner's article is a fairly typical example of mainstream media transphobia. If we unpick the central argument of her piece, we get closer to understanding where such myths and intolerance stem from.

Turner opens her piece by explaining to the reader why, in her opinion, Travis is wrong:

Travis Alabanza is a performance artist who, in the tradition of Leigh Bowery, Boy George or Bowie, dresses to astonish and

---

1 www.thetimes.co.uk/article/children-sacrificed-to-appease-trans-lobby-bqom2mm95 (last accessed 02/2019).

subvert. Blue lipstick, beard stubble, fab shoes, frocks, mad hair, attitude. What Travis isn't, however, is a woman.

Travis explicitly states their pronoun is them. Yet Turner misgenders Travis repeatedly throughout the article. What does it mean when Turner claims to be right? It suggests that while Travis is either deceiving us about who they are, or indeed lying to themselves, Turner, on the other hand, embodies the full expression of authenticity. Turner believes that she has access to 'realness', while Travis is defined by superficiality, and her view is underpinned by the debates from the previous chapter that say that gender is biological and essential and anyone that deviates from that binary is therefore unnatural.

Turner is not alone: pronouns are a hot topic for the right. Misgendering and trans rights are used as a way in to rail about free speech, political correctness, the so-called snowflake generation and the left. What we're witnessing here, in the words of 'J', a 22-year-old trans man and activist, is intentional, aggressive and repeated misgendering:,

'J', 22

I never felt right in the body I was born in. For a lot of my childhood and early adolescence I thought I was a lesbian, but it took me until my late teens to feel comfortable enough to tell my friends and family who I am: that I'm a man. Being trans has got easier the older I've become. I could not be more grateful to those around me who have shown me so much understanding and support from such a young age. I know it wasn't easy, especially for my parents.

The online abuse has been awful, and it has seriously affected my mental health. I'm much better now, but for a while I was having daily panic attacks and even thought about ending my life. I've had every name you could possibly imagine thrown at me. This kind of abuse is very different from people accidentally calling me 'she' or a girl. Personally, I really don't mind that so much: it's just about giving me the respect and listening to me when I correct you.

'It's just a phase'

As Turner states, rates of people in the UK seeking support to transition have risen in recent years. She puts the blame on what she calls a 'trans lobby', who are committing 'child abuse' by encouraging and supporting young people to transition, who come to regret their decision in later years.

Turner is right: there has been a rise of young people seeking medical support to transition, or support from NHS mental health services to talk through their experiences. I spoke to Nicky Ryan, the co-founder of Free2B Alliance, an organisation based in South London that gives support to young LGBTQ+ people. In her words:

I've definitely seen an increase in number of young people accessing support. What's so wrong is that the media portrays this as if being trans is a phase and as if they are pushed into it. This is so far from the truth. What people don't see is that these young people have been battling and struggling for a very long time, and that today – with all the new brilliant TV shows – young people people are saying 'okay! That's me! I can finally be who I am.' I know a lot of people worry about kids being pushed into it but that's just not the case. No one can be forced into transitioning.

I think people worry that children will transition and then change their minds. Personally, I've been working in the industry for over 20 years and I have not met a single person that that's happened to.

It's not just Turner who believes that being trans is an adolescent phase. Melanie McDonagh for the *Evening Standard* wrote 'the notion that you can simply put on a gender the way you change your contact lenses is, I think, symptomatic of a worrying indifference to a basic question of what makes us ourselves.'[2]

Unsurprisingly, Turner did not interview any trans people for her article. If she had, she would have learned that gender is not something that you can jump around in. You can't pick up a gender in the morning like you would a pair of socks or shoes – in a utopia this might be the case, but it's not the world we live in today. People lose their families over being trans; are shut out of work; face bullying and harassment; undergo an invasive, dehumanising and often traumatic process of legally changing their sex; and then there's the fear of being 'outed', of not passing, of having their body looked at with suspicion, people trying to find 'proof' of their dishonesty and deceit. In my experience, changing contact lenses is nothing like this. Part of the reason so many more young people are seeking support for their gender identity is because of the important national conversation that's being led by trans and gender non-conforming people, like Travis.

The law

Turner accuses Travis of being a danger to society:

They are just permitting men – any man – to walk into a flimsily curtained space where giggling teenage girls check out

---

2   www.standard.co.uk/comment/comment/melanie-mcdonagh-changing-sex-is-not-to-be-done-just-on-a-whim-a3149031.html (last accessed 02/2019).

a friend's new dress in their bras. Topshop's female customers were baffled. Why sacrifice our privacy and safety?

The stereotype that trans people are a threat is not uncommon; it came to the fore most perniciously during debates about a consultation to amend the UK's 2004 Gender Recognition Act.

At the time of writing, it is possible in the UK to change your legal gender after you have proved two things: a) you have been living in your preferred gender for at least two years and b) that you are suffering from 'gender dysphoria'. Many trans activists and allies have argued that this process is dehumanising, lengthy and intrusive. Currently 'gender dysphoria' is a recognised mental health condition, the implication being that if you want to change gender you have to say that you're sick. Providing you have met the medical criteria, you can then be considered by a panel that will decide to believe you (or not) and then warrant your legal recognition. The potential changes to the Act will simply streamline this process, but they were met with rage nonetheless. A group of Trans Exclusionary Radical Feminists (TERFS) were so furious that they staged a protest, storming an all-male swimming pool on Hampstead Heath, London, wearing fake beards.

When the consultation took place, the debate boiled down to accessing single gender spaces like toilets, rape crisis centres, prisons and changing rooms. TERFs and other critics argued that the changes will mean that predatory men will pretend to be trans women so they can enter these spaces and prey on vulnerable people. In the words of Turner, '[Topshop] are just permitting men – any man – to walk into a flimsily curtained space where giggling teenage girls check out a friend's new dress in their bras.' The debates also took place at the same time as the highly publicised sexual assaults of Karen White, a 52-year-old trans women who was imprisoned in New Hall prison in West Yorkshire and sexually assaulted two female inmates. The question of trans rights and sexual violence therefore becomes inextricably linked in mainstream discourses.

For some commentators challenging sexual violence means ensuring that trans women do not access safe spaces, such as domestic violence shelters. Every single day in England and Wales alone, there are approximately 1,400 sexual assaults by men on women. Two women are killed each week by a current or former partner in England and Wales and 90 per cent of violent crime is committed by men.[3] Behind every single statistic is a person: the scale of sexual and gender violence is devastating and we would all agree that it needs to be tackled.

The argument rests on the idea that people assigned male (i.e. having a penis, higher levels of testosterone and testes) have the propensity to be more dangerous and violent and therefore need to be kept away from vulnerable women. Clearly it's a highly emotive topic for many – however, there is absolutely no evidence at all that trans women are a particularly violent group in society.[4] In the words of Ruth Hall, Chief Executive of Stonewall charity, 'much of this coverage has focused on particularly emotive issues – whether based on evidence or not.'

If we look at the facts, it's trans women themselves that are subjected to some of the greatest violence than any community in society. Trans survivors are also one of the most hidden groups of domestic abuse survivors.[5] In Stonewall's research around the UK they found that domestic violence organisations have been supporting trans women for a long time and that that support is

---

3 www.ons.gov.uk/peoplepopulationandcommunity/crimeandjustice/compendium/focusonviolentcrimeandsexualoffences/yearendingmarch2015/chapter2homicide.

4 www.stonewall.org.uk/sites/default/files/stonewall_and_nfpsynergy_report.pdf.

5 http://safelives.org.uk/sites/default/files/resources/LGBT%2B%20NSP%20Report.pdf.

vital because one in six trans women have faced domestic violence in the last twelve months.[6]

Why is it always trans women who are the focus of such scrutiny in the media's eye and not trans men? Is it because they chose to let go of their male privilege and become a woman? In *Whipping Girl*, Julia Serano says: 'most of the anti-trans sentiment that I have had to deal with as a transsexual woman is probably better described as misogyny'.[7] She coined the term transmisogyny to explain this phenomenon, showing that it rests on *both* transphobia and misogyny, and the assumption that masculinity is in all ways superior to femininity. For trans women and gender non-conforming people of colour, like Travis, transmisogyny compounds with racism. We know that these women experience some of the worst and most brutal forms of violence than any other group in society – interpersonal violence, institutional violence, state sanctioned violence and sexual violence.

Serano's concept of transmisogyny helps explain *why* commentators are so preoccupied with this law change – because in reality the Act will not lead to any changes of gender segregated spaces at all. According to the Equality Act 2010, all trans people who have undergone, are undergoing or intend to undergo gender transition – even if they don't have legal recognition – are *already* allowed to access women-only spaces. As research by Stonewall and many others shows, trans women have been accessing women's toilets and crisis centres for decades.

Whose safety have we prioritised? Rather than pushing the interests of cis people to the front and centre, let's ask another question: how does society pose a threat to trans people?

- 80 per cent of young trans people have self-harmed

---

6 www.stonewall.org.uk/sites/default/files/stonewall_and_nfpsynergy_report.pdf.
7 Julia Serano, *Whipping Girl: A Transsexual Woman on Sexism and the Scapegoating of Femininity* (New York: Basic Books, 2007), 12.

- 40 per cent of young trans people have attempted suicide[8]
- Two in five trans people (41 per cent) and three in ten non-binary people (31 per cent) have experienced a hate crime of incident because of their gender identity in the past twelve months[9]
- One in four trans people have experienced homelessness at some point in their lives[10]
- One in eight trans people (12 per cent) have been physically attacked by colleagues or customers in the past twelve months[11]

The discrimination and violence against gender non-conforming people is inextricably linked to conditions of poverty, the mental health crisis engulfing young generations and to the closure and resource depletion of support services.

Supporting our own

While there are without a doubt toxic and vocal subsections of society who are outwardly and proudly transphobic, and a large number who simply through their own lack of experience are misinformed, there is also a growing movement of understanding, tolerance and resistance. When I spoke to Nicky Ryan from Free2B, she was keen to emphasize how much had changed in the attitudes of young people, and how hopeful she was. Schools in the UK are increasingly including trans rights on their curriculums, gender neutral toilets are becoming more common; and activists and public figures like model Monroe Bergorf, Travis Alabanza,

8 Stonewall School Report 2017.

9 LGBT in Britain: Trans Report (London: Stonewall, 2018) www.stonewall.org.uk/system/files/lgbt_in_britain_-_trans_report_final.pdf.

10 Ibid.

11 https://broadly.vice.com/en_us/article/43q8pj/one-in-eight-transgender-people-uk-physically-attacked-work.

actress Laverne Cox and YouTuber Jaz Jennings, among many others, have opened up space for understanding, support and resilience. Rather than shaming and denying the agency of gender non-conforming people, cis people must act in solidarity. In the words of Yoyo, a 20-year-old student from Hong Kong:

Yoyo, 20

My dad is a trans woman and I am from Hong Kong, which is still a very traditional place. It was really tough at first. However Dad said she felt like a woman all her life so I don't think there's any reasonable way for me to ignore her feelings. Obviously I accepted her, it would be paternalistic to presume you know why someone would decide who they are.

I had to do a lot of research when my Dad came out. I was ten, and at that point the most you've seen about gender identity is when the prince kissed the princess on Disney. For me my Dad is a female. And it's like okay . . . what does that mean? Why does she cross dress? What even is a woman? After you get over the 'my parents are really mad' and 'why are they always shouting', I came to a point of acceptance where I could say: okay, my dad is a woman. And why does she like my mum another woman? Right, so women can like women! That's when I started desperately Googling at ten 'women liking women' . . . I came across some very inappropriate sites and it's actually how I learned about porn.

There is no right way to be a woman. The ultimate rule is that you can be a woman if you want to be a woman. If you are a woman you are a woman. You're not a woman if you are demure, submissive, you can cook and you can bake. Or if you have breasts or a vagina. There are enough pressures in the world without us supporting our own people.

Chapter 3

Masculinity: Trump's button

In 2005 Donald Trump was recorded having this conversation with TV host Billy Bush:

> Trump: I better use some Tic Tacs just in case I start kissing her. You know I'm automatically attracted to beautiful . . . I just start kissing them. It's like a magnet. Just kiss. I don't even wait. And when you're a star, they let you do it. You can do anything.
>
> Bush: Whatever you want?
>
> Trump: Absolutely. Grab them by the pussy.

The video was released by the *Washington Post* in 2016, just days before an important presidential debate between Trump and Hillary Clinton. In an attempt to defend himself against the onslaught of criticism, Trump said that he was 'embarrassed' but that it was 'locker room talk' and 'it's just one of those things'.

The recording swiftly gained international notoriety. The question many asked was: what even is locker room talk and why is it a get out of jail free card? Trump's defence rested on an assumption that when men are behind closed doors, away from the watchful eyes of women and the wider world, they are bound by solidarity; it is in these moments that men can speak honestly and freely. Aside from the fact that, clearly, a lot of men do not talk about women like this (not all men are even attracted to women), Trump does not keep these kinds of conversations private. He makes a point about being as public as possible. He speaks openly about assaulting women, he proudly insults the way women look and he gloats in front of a world audience about the size of both his penis and nuclear button respectively: his masculinity is worn like a badge blazing on his sleeve for all to see.

Trump took a gamble. He believed that not only would people not care about him saying these things, but that presenting himself as an exaggerated alpha male would help his campaign. In the end he was right. 62,984,825 people turned up to the polling station to vote for him and on 8 November 2016 he became the President-elect.[1] Now that he's safely installed in the White House, Trump continues to beat his chest and his approval ratings have remained relatively steady, with somewhere between 35–38 per cent of Americans standing behind him. Trump also has international support. Among British populations, YouGov polls show that he is the seventh most popular politician in the world.[2] It's not uncommon to see Trump masks at a far-right demo, but as this poll clearly shows, it's not just extremists that view him as a good leader.

Obviously, Trump will leave office at some point, but when that moment happens, what kind of politics will be left behind? No matter how hard liberal commentators have tried to define his electoral success as a freak occurrence, it simply doesn't look that way. Trump was a symptom of something far more structural and global. While history tells us that there are plenty of causes that explain a rise in fascism – economic crisis and scapegoating, for instance – gender is one essential part of the story. It has been

---

1   https://edition.cnn.com/election/2016/results/president.
2   https://yougov.co.uk/topics/international/explore/public_figure/Donald_Trump.

called 'a dangerous rush of testosterone' and the modern crisis in masculinity.[3] Outdated ideals about what it means to be a man have led to the election of a string of alpha males to run the world today, from Brazil's Jair Bolsonaro, to India's Narendra Modi, to Turkey's Recep Erdoğan.

Here, we're going to look mostly at masculinity. In Chapter 7, we'll look more at femininity, virginity and purity.

The warrior: Strength, might and power

Only a man who knows what it is like to be defeated can reach down to the bottom of his soul and come up with the extra ounce of power it takes to win when the match is even. – Muhammad Ali

'Gendered expression' ranges from the most ostensibly minute incident – how we sit down in a chair, to the way our hair looks and the way we talk – all the way to more profound patterns of behaviour, such as how we relate to others. Masculinity and femininity are the qualities that are associated with what it means, in a traditional sense, to be a man or woman. As we've seen, these qualities are often assumed to be determined by someone's sex, but in reality they are much more fragile.

Strength, might and power have long been fundamental components of masculinity; what's changed is what we understand strength, might and power to look like. Take colour, for instance. Today there are rigid ideas about pink and blue, the former being a symbol of femininity and the latter of masculinity. But the idea that pink is somehow 'unmanly' is a relatively new notion. In the eighteenth century, it was considered the height of fashion for men to wear a flowery pink suit. Right up into the 1920s pink was

---

3   www.theguardian.com/books/2018/mar/17/the-crisis-in-modern-masculinity (last accessed 02/2019).

seen as a strong working class male colour linked to 'being in the pink', in other words having flushed cheeks and a healthy composition. Similarly, in some cultures, having your ears pierced is a right of passage for young girls, but seen on men is a symbol of effeminateness or being gay. In some punk communities, having a piercing signals strength and a resilience to pain, the most stereotypical masculine qualities. In England skirts are seen as feminine, but in India it is common to see men wearing the skirt-like Lungi, or kilt in Scotland. The examples are endless.

Gendered expectations of character have also changed. When the British Empire was booming in the eighteenth and early nineteenth centuries, those characteristics closely associated to the military and nation building came to define the ideals of English manliness. In the eighteenth century in England though, men who engaged in acts of violence – against women, other men and children – or indeed participated in 'blood sports', like bare-knuckle boxing matches, were considered the idealised embodiment of virility. The masculine virtues of adventure, risk-taking and danger were elevated, and the qualities associated with women were denigrated.[4] It might seem farfetched for a reader today, but, even in such a hyper-masculine Georgian society, it was not seen as effeminate when men talked about their feelings. On the contrary, it was actually thought that the most refined and manly men had strong emotions that erupted, uncontrollably, from time to time.

It would take explicitly counter-Enlightenment thinkers in the eighteenth century to put forward anti-racist and feminist views of humanity. Victorian values of manhood and race fermented in all male spaces: in pubs, coffeehouses, the pews of Protestant churches and the classrooms of the English public school system. The values of being a good father, providing for the family, being

---

4   David Morgan, 'Class and Masculinity,' in *Handbook of Studies on Men and Masculinities*, eds. S. Michael Kimmel, Jeff Hearn and R.W. Connell (New York: Sage Publications, 2005), 169.

measured, chivalrous, protective of women, and exhibiting self-control, physical endurance and courage prevailed among the upper classes. Emotional men were no longer in vogue and with Britain now being the global leading power, Eton became a training ground for world governance.

You might wonder why Victorian values still matter today. But when we look at who holds power around the world, it looks on the surface like very little has changed. Globally, the 0.0001 per cent – the richest and most powerful six to seven thousand people in the world – are 94 per cent male, overwhelmingly white and mostly from North America and Europe. The institutions that set the world's agenda have changed: where there was once the East India Company and the British Crown, we now have G8 (now the G7 after the exclusion of Russia), G20, NATO, the World Bank, the IMF and the World Trade Organisation.[5] But if we're looking at the individuals who are deemed capable of ruling, the comparison to the nineteenth century is damning.

A performance

More often than not, those people we imagine as the ultimate expression of masculinity are removed from us. Be that Trump, Mike Tyson, Arnold Schwarzenegger or an ancient Greek statue, they tend to be celebrities, historical or mythological characters. When it comes to men in our lives, do they actually fulfil the ideal of masculinity?

Ola

I find it strange that strength is seen as an exclusively masculine quality. When I look around me I see men and women debunking this idea all the time. I'm aware that a lot of men

5   David Rothkopf, *Superclass: The Global Power Elite and the World They are Making* (London: Little, Brown, 2008).

treat their female partners like unpaid therapists in private while appearing indestructible in public. The idea that men are inherently strong is just not true – we are pretending to be strong. We don't choose to be men. Most men – myself included – learn to put on this performance when we're young.

Scratch the surface and masculinity is revealed to be like a towering and illusive institution that's impossible to live up to – and very easy to crash around you. This is clear when, as Ola states, we actually interrogate the relationships in our lives and see that it's not always cis-men who display the most character-istically masculine attributes. But it's also evident that while the pressures of gender are ever so present, they can also topple down out of our control.

Heterosexual virility was a cornerstone of masculine ideals long before Trump's mine-is-bigger-than-yours demeanour. The classicist Jean-Paul Thuillier notes that the word virile stems from the Latin, *virilitas*, which could refer quite simply to the 'male organs'. While the expectation of sexual performance is at the heart of the masculine ideal, it is a fragile aspiration. While erectile dysfunction (ED, also known as impotence) is often associated with ageing, that's not the whole picture. Approximately 40 per cent of men are affected at age 40 and nearly 70 per cent of men are affected at age 70, however approximately one in four people under the age of 40 have sought medical treatment for it at one point in their lives.[6,7] It's an extremely common medical condition – beyond an individual's control – that directly challenges the masculine ideal.[8]

---

6   www.huffpost.com/entry/erectile-dysfunction-young-men-age-40-younger_n_3405085.

7   H. A. Feldman, I. Goldstein, D. G. Hatzichristou, R. J. Krane and J. B. McKinlay, 'Impotence and its medical and psychosocial correlates: Results of the Massachusetts Male Aging Study,' *J Urol* 151, (1994): 54–61.

8   American Psychiatric Association, *Diagnostic and Statistical Manual of Mental Disorders*, fifth edition (Washington, DC: American Psychiatric Association, 2013).

Masculine ideals have also long been associated with work. In spite of the expectation that the male of the household should be the main breadwinner, this pressure is fragile and subjected to shocks from outside ourselves. In an already deeply unequal and classed British society, harsh austerity measures have resulted in mass redundancies, mass job losses, mass homelessness and deepening precarious employment across the country. Austerity has hit women and in particular women of colour the hardest, but as many academics have shown, these structural economic problems have also had a devastating effect on the mental health of men. The economic disempowerment directly challenges what is supposed to be 'a real man' and the devastating effect of these impossible standards on men is clear.[9,10]

Job losses, unemployment and precariousness have an effect on mental health. The most recent figures show the northeast of England has the highest avoidable mortality rate for males in the country, with suicide at the second highest rate in the UK. For many commentators, this bears some relation to the fact that this area had the joint-lowest average actual weekly hours of work by men during the last tax year. Clearly there's an important class element to masculinity and work here. Shockwaves from the 2008 financial crisis were not absorbed by the upper classes – it was the poorest in society that took the largest burden, with even many in the middle classes also taking a hit.

Masculinity in excess

In 2014, the London School of Economics (LSE) rugby club disbanded after some of its members were caught handing out a flyer at Fresher's Fair, trying to draw new first year recruits

---

9   www.ons.gov.uk/peoplepopulationandcommunity/healthandsocialcare/causesofdeath/bulletins/avoidablemortalityinenglandandwales/2015.

10   www.intersecting-inequalities.com.

into the club. The content of the flyer was a garbled cliché of lad culture, misogyny and homophobia. Women were called 'mingers', 'trollops' and 'slags' and girls who play sports 'beast-like'. There were comments about not tolerating 'outright homosexual debauchery' in addition to identifying students at the 'poly' (polytechnic university) 'scum' who will 'all work for us one day'.

In excess, the masculine qualities of boldness, courage, resilience and strength of mind become aggressiveness, violence and chauvinism. Couple this with the power of class privilege that many at universities like LSE possess and lad culture becomes toxic. This is no new phenomenon. For a select few, the 1960s and 1970s was a time of wild hedonism and sexual permissiveness. Rock stars were known for sleeping with streams of women and for having entourages of groupies who would travel far and wide to get it on with their heroes. There's nothing wrong with sleeping around, but the way they speak about women reveals the kind of entitlement that is reminiscent of the LSE rugby club. One of Elvis Presley's entourage, Lamar Fike, told *Mojo* magazine, 'Elvis gets more ass than a toilet seat. Six girls in the room at one time . . . when we left places it took the national guard to clean things up'.[11] Or, as John Lennon later told *Rolling Stone* magazine, 'If you could get on our tours, you were in . . . Wherever we were there was always a whole scene going on. [Hotel rooms] full of junk and whores and fuck knows what.'[12]

The fantasy of male strength measures itself most gratifyingly against the fantasy of female weakness. – Pankaj Mishra

Traditional masculinity and femininity are like Yin and Yang; binary and oppositional but also complimentary. Where men are

---

11 Mick Wall, *When Giants Walked the Earth* (London: Orion Publishing Group, 2008).
12 Ibid.

supposed to have physical strength, women should be physically soft. Where men have cool logic, women are emotional. The positive qualities of femininity, such as gentleness, kindness and empathy, are thought of in opposition to the greater excesses of masculinity. And vice versa. The weaknesses of femininity, such as passivity and neurosis are balanced out by decisiveness and cool-headedness. Within this idea of gender relations, the hetero-sexual couple – man and woman or husband and wife – reigns supreme, as the most harmonious and most peaceful way to organise society.

These seemingly abstract reflections on how masculinity and femininity are put against each other have real life consequences. After England football matches – which for all their undeniable collective joy are also extremely masculine spaces – domestic violence shelters and charities register a radical spike in the number of instances of gendered violence. Journal of Research in Crime and Delinquency, reported that instances rose by 38 per cent when the England team lost a game and by 26 per cent when the team won or drew. This doesn't just apply to football: research-ers found that men were 10 per cent more likely to use violence against their female partner if their team lost an American National Football League game.[13]

But masculinity in excess also hurts men:

- Men are half as likely as women to visit their GP[14]
- British women are more likely to be anxious and depressed, and more likely to attempt suicide but men are three times more likely than women to be successful and take their own lives
- The rate of premature deaths (under 50 years) is one and a half times higher among men than women. This is primarily

---

due to cardiovascular disease, accidents, suicide and cancer. All of which are preventable with the right medical attention[15]

Max, 23

I don't ever talk to my male friends about anything. Like if a friend goes on a date, all we would ask is did you have sex. And then we'll be like was she peng. Then he might show us a photo of her on Instagram and we'll be like ye she's peng. That's it.

Ola

I think about masculinity all of the time. I think about all of the male friends I've lost because they acted in a way that I found stifling – whether that was because they weren't emotionally well-rounded, which made it really hard to be able to talk openly about our feelings; they did something awful (usually to women) or because I felt like they were in competition with me.

I think about the number of times I've been sexually harassed by white women – in clubs, at University, house parties – my white ex who had jungle fever, and the insecure black men who acquiesce to sexual racism. I'm reminded of this video online of a black man who telling his male friends that he had been raped by a woman while crying and also laughing at the same time. All of his friends were also laughing along. But this guy was trying to explain to his friends how bad he felt, and the only way they could talk about it was through banter. Something similar happened to me and when I explained the situation to a female friend – a seemingly switched on white liberal – she laughed.

---

15   www.poverty.org.uk/60/index.shtml.

As Ola explains, the threat of being called feminine – due to expressing what you might think of as 'feminine' traits – can be used to undermine and degrade men. Whereas traditional masculinity is aggressively heterosexual, male homosexuality is typically associated with effeminateness. Words like 'poof', 'gay', 'homo' are as much about emasculation as they are about sexuality. Within the gay male community in the UK, one study found that 69 per cent of men said that they had been made to feel like less of a man because of their sexuality.[16]

Feminine qualities are also ascribed to groups of men as a means to Other and create an enemy. Pankaj Mishra argues that throughout the nineteenth century, increasingly fixed gender roles had an impact on men of colour beyond European borders. Its most insidious expression was the conquest and exploitation of people deemed feminine, and, therefore, less than human – a violence that became normalised in the nineteenth century. For many Europeans and Americans, to be a true man was to be an ardent imperialist and nationalist. Such imperialist projects rested on the idea that since 'other' men were more feminine, they were not only easy to crush, but they needed to be wiped away. Exactly the same notion of masculinity was adopted by German forces, 'Weakness must be eliminated' said Hitler during his years in power. Jews, disabled people, those with mental health conditions or learning difficulties were all represented as effeminate, as deviations from a pure and idealised form of Aryan masculinity.

Masculinity in excess entrenches the binary between feminine and masculine. But as we've seen such rigid thinking does not hold up to scrutiny. The binary might be false, but it has very real and tangible consequences – both on individuals, but also as we're seeing today in the wider political area. Much like the imperial leaders of the nineteenth century, many of the newly elected far

16   https://attitude.co.uk/attitudes-masculinity-survey-reveals-75-of-gay-men-are-turned-off-by-effeminate-guys.

right have declared a war on weakness. But we have to ask the question of how stable they actually are. Trump may build a wall around America, but what kind of instability does that unleash on families that live around the border? Bolsonaro, leader of Brazil, who famously said 'Yes, I'm homophobic – and very proud of it,' calls into question the safety of the LGBTQ community. In what world can that ever be called stable leadership?[17]

17   www.theguardian.com/world/2018/oct/27/dispatch-sao-paulo-jair-bolsonaro-victory-lgbt-community-fear.

45

Chapter 4

Body image: From scrawny to brawny

Khin, 23[1]

I have very good body image. I adore every part of my physical being and I love being naked. There are days when I wish I had bigger boobs, a bigger booty, and thicker eyebrows – social media is definitely the main source of those insecurities – but at the end of the day, I feel very happy.

Khin is an exception . . . the overwhelming majority of people are wracked by imagined physical failings. How did we get here? Did Neanderthals roam the earth agonising about thigh gaps? Did cavemen lie awake at night dreaming of the good life with a smaller nose?

Thousands of years of documented history show that there has always been an idea of who or what is beautiful. In Ancient Greek mythology, the dazzling looks of Helen, the wife of Menelaus, King of Sparta, were a weapon of mass destruction. The legend goes that the Goddess of Love and Beauty, Aphrodite, promised Paris the most beautiful woman in the world, so he set out from Troy to abduct Helen. Her beauty, the saying goes, 'launched a thousand

---

1   Many of the names in this book have been changed.

ships' because when Menelaus realised Helen was missing he mobilised an army and started the Trojan War.

But what did the most beautiful woman in history look like?[2] A typical Spartan Queen from 3,000 years ago would have worn thick black eye make-up, she would have had sun-like tattoos covering her entire face and an almost entirely shaven head, aside from a few remaining strands carefully sculpted to look like snakes.

Today, Helen's punk-like look might do it for some but she's a million miles from a typical Victoria's Secret model. What this tells us is important: that while beauty standards have always existed, they are in flux and are subject to change. Examining them can tell us something about the values of the time.

The beauty myth

Naomi Shimada is admired as one of the most exciting models in the world. At 30, with around 80,000 followers on Instagram, she has become a figure of resistance within the fashion industry for challenging rigid beauty norms. Naomi is UK size 16, which makes her average for the western world, but in the fashion industry she is considered 'plus'.

Naomi is loud and open about most of the challenging aspects of the fashion industry, stories that are far from unusual. 'As a model, dieting is what's always on your mind – it completely takes over your life and it's all you can talk and think about. You can't just have breakfast and eat bacon and laugh because you're hating yourself all the time.'[3] Things are changing however, and Naomi

---

2 When I talk about 'women' throughout the book, I am referring to anyone who identifies as a woman – cis, intersex or trans. The same goes for 'man' or 'men'. More on gender in Chapters 2, 3 and 4.

3 www.theguardian.com/global/2015/oct/18/naomi-shimada-why-plus-is-a-dirty-word-in-fashion.

is at the forefront of challenging the representation of women in the media.

Arguably the most important book on body image is Naomi Wolf's hugely influential *The Beauty Myth*, published in 1990. Wolf showed how the beauty industry – in fashion, advertising and magazines – erased difference, and forged a very specific, narrow type of femininity. Wolf argued that with the advancement of some women in the middle of the twentieth century, daunting and unattainable beauty standards emerged that made most women feel inadequate. Sure, there have always been certain expectations and unwritten rules about the ways that women feel they should look – take a walk around any gallery stocked with Renaissance art and that becomes evident – but what changed was the extreme and unprecedented pressure to conform. 'The Beauty Myth', according to Wolf, was a method of social control. Where women were once worried about the dishes piling up, they now transferred guilt to their looks.[4]

Wolf showed that these expectations were everywhere, but they were especially prevalent in women's magazines. The number of articles about dieting rose by 70 per cent in women's magazines from 1968 to 1972.[5] Wolf argues that these articles have a deeply negative effect on the reader's self-esteem. She interviews one woman who said that buying women's magazines for her was a 'form of self-abuse': 'Yes! Wow! I can be better starting right from this minute! Look at her! Look at her! Right afterward, I feel like throwing out all my clothes and everything in my refrigerator and telling my boyfriend never to call me again and blowtorching my whole life.' This may sound familiar. A study by Bradley University in Illinois found that just three minutes looking at fashion

---

4 Naomi Wolf, *The Beauty Myth: How Images of Beauty are Used Against Women* (London: Vintage, 1991).

5 Ibid., 128.

magazines led to 70 per cent of women feeling 'guilty, depressed and shameful'.[6]

As Wolf articulates, these magazines packaged up and sold just one kind of femininity. When she was writing in the 1990s, and when I was growing up, it was the controversial 'waif' or 'heroin chic' look we were taught to aspire to, typified by Kate Moss and other top models who had bodies that resembled those of pre-pubescent children. They were almost exclusively white, underweight, cis and able bodied and while of course many people do naturally have that kind of body type, the waif look was sold as a meritocratic fantasy that we could all attain, just like any other distant dream of self-improvement. Work out enough, diet enough, work hard enough at your job, at school and you can have it all. The truth was stark – the vast majority of us will never be heroin chic, just as we will never be impossibly rich.

The waif emerged during a time of extremes. Extreme global inequality in 1990 meant that at a time when around one billion people were starving, humans around the world were on average getting larger and larger. In the 1990s, the World Health Organisation (WHO) sounded the alarm for the first time about a global obesity epidemic.[7] It was within this context that fashion models were getting smaller and smaller. The trend peaked in 2009 when Kate Moss revealed her professional and life motto: 'Nothing tastes as good as skinny feels'. This declaration resonated so profoundly and was so controversial because there was an element of truth to it. Skinniness was not just about looks – it had come to be about the only desirable, the only moral; the only acceptable way to *be*.

6   E. Stice and H. E. Shaw, 'Adverse Effects of the Media Portrayed Thin-Ideal on Women and Linkages to Bulimic Symptomatology,' *Journal of Social and Clinical Psychology* (1994), quoted by The Body Project study by the Women's Studies Program of Bradley University (2012).
7   The World Bank. (2016). Retrieved from www.worldbank.org/en/topic/poverty/overview. Accessed September 2018.

Riots not diets

Since the 1990s, cultural icons have changed and so have beauty standards. Where once it was all about Kate Moss, Sienna Miller and Jennifer Aniston, now Beyonce, the Kardashians and Naomi Shimada have taken centre stage. Naomi agreed with this. 'Things have got better. There are some extraordinary people taking the lead to change beauty representations from within the industry'.

The body positivity movement is in full swing. So-called plus-size model Ashley Graham has even had a Barbie doll made in her image. By Graham's request, the doll's thighs even touch. Models that speak out about being told to 'lose weight' in the fashion industry are celebrated and have seen their careers blossom.

Centuries old Western beauty norms around race mean that white women have dominated beauty magazines, fashion runways, film, TV and most forms of media. For years, Bristol model Naomi Campbell would be one of the few women of colour in high end fashion, and in 1997 she spoke out about it when she told an interviewer that 'there is prejudice. It is a problem and I can't go along any more with brushing it under the carpet.' Later that year, she attacked the 'narrow-mindedness' of a newsstand culture in which 'this business is about selling, and blond and blue-eyed girls are what sells'.[8] Today, however, just like we have witnessed greater diversity around weight and body shape, there's also far more racial diversity on runways and in the fashion industry as a whole. In Autumn 2018's fashion weeks around the world, 32.5 per cent were catwalk models of colour, in comparison to 17 per cent just three years earlier in 2015. Clearly, it doesn't go far enough – but there are obvious trends in the right direction. In 2018 there were also more trans, intersex and non-binary models on the runway than ever before.

---

8   www.theguardian.com/fashion/2017/oct/16/naomi-campbell-naomissance-top-of-fashion-world (last accessed 01/2019).

Media and fashion have responded to outcries from grassroots body positive movements to stop peddling impossible beauty standards and to reflect the variety of human bodies. This is being led in part by the new economic and political power that social media platforms such as Instagram hold. Since the 1990s, magazine sales have plummeted, and power has shifted away from the publishing houses to decentralised social media platforms like Instagram, which at the time of writing has over one billion users. Informed by the politics of LGBTQ+, feminist and anti-racism movements, among others, Instagram users proudly use hashtags like #bodypositive, #SaggyBoobsMatter #honourmycurves #blackgirlmagic #thickthighs #transisbeautiful adorn people's home-feeds. For all the negative press that social media gets – much of it rightly – body positive activism online has been empowering and genuinely life changing for some.

Saff, 21

I grew up in a small village and my family were the only brown Muslim people that we knew. Our community was isolated and insular. I watched porn when I was young, and I did start to have very negative perceptions about my body. I was so insecure about my vulva. I was like oh my god my labia! What's wrong with it! It was always things I had no control over. I'm brown so I'm quite hairy. Everyone around me was white and had fair hair. I hated having hair. I had experiences where people would call me monkey aged about six because I had quite dark hair on my legs and arms. Tumblr was the only place that I was exposed to a whole different world. It helped me more than anything else. I am so grateful that I can now detach myself from expectations of how I'm supposed to look.

I spoke to disability rights activist and academic, Kush Westwood, about her experience with online body positive activism:

There is such a huge range of experiences with disabilities that it would be impossible to make any kind of sweeping statement about all disabled people. Personally, I have hyper mobility syndrome so I have always had dislocations during sex, which is appalling, really. There's a real problem with what people think is body-normal, especially given that most people get their sex education from porn and mass produced porn in particular. The kinds of bodies most people think is normal is absolutely not the range of normal. Of course that's enormously anxiety inducing for a lot of people. For much of my youth I felt like my body was completely out of the norm and it's only since I've encountered body positive activists who've said 'no your body is okay' that I've come to a place of acceptance. All humans have a range of bodies and there is no such thing as the right body. I only wish someone had told me that at the age of sixteen. My life would have been a lot easier.

On to pastures new

In 1971, Coca-Cola released one of its most famous adverts. A crowd of people from around the world, all wearing traditional dress, were filmed on a hill in Italy holding bottles of coke and singing 'I'd Like to Buy the World a Coke', a jingle about spreading peace, love and joy by buying the world's favourite fizzy drink. It was widely criticised for co-opting and profiting from the values of liberation and peace that the 1960s movements had fought for.

The body positivity movement started online as a radical demand, but much like the Coca Cola advert, it is no longer uncommon to see the ideals echoed by brands around the world. Zara took a stab at it with their 'love your curves' campaign, depicting two very slim blonde women as poster girls. Victoria's Secret were lambasted for their 'Perfect Body' poster, depicting eight very pale skinned and underweight models, ultimately they caved into the pressure and changed their slogan to 'a body for everybody'. Should you wish you can even buy, for a mere $710, a highly subversive Dior T-Shirt saying 'We should all be feminists', after Chimamanda Ngozi Adichie's 2014 book on feminism for the modern day.

Where there's societal changes, there's also an opportunity to make money. In the words of a journalist writing for *Forbes* magazine, 'Non-Caucasian women represent a real sweet spot in today's market. Ad campaigns like those for Glossier and Cover Girl include models of different ages, ethnicities and body types'.[9]

All research shows that when we have low self-esteem we spend more money on our appearance. The amount of money the average woman in the UK spends on her appearance is already a massive £70,294 in a lifetime.[10] That's £1,352 a year or £112.65 a month.[11] Instagram has replaced magazines as the primary media for advertising campaigns, with influencers paid tens of thousands of pounds to promote certain products and brands on their feed. There's more regulation now, and influencers have to indicate where they're in a 'paid partnership' with a brand or company. But this doesn't stop the incessant bombardment of sponsored content. There is an enormous commercial incentive to ensure we continue to be dissatisfied with our bodies.

A decade after Moss' mantra and it is now passé for fashion models to admit to starvation, but does that mean there are no beauty standards or that the pressures of commercialisation have halted? Sadly not. In 2018 *Love Island*, ITV2's most watched

---

9 www.forbes.com/sites/michaelrsolomon/2018/06/07/fashion-marketers-who-is-beautiful-hint-not-just-reese-witherspoon/#39809fee26bb (last accessed 02/2019).

10 www.independent.co.uk/life-style/fashion/average-british-woman-spend-70000-appearance-lifetime-cosmetics-beauty-products-groupon-uk-a7623201.html (last accessed 01/2019).

11 www.independent.co.uk/life-style/fashion/average-british-woman-spend-70000-appearance-lifetime-cosmetics-beauty-products-groupon-uk-a7623201.html (last accessed 01/2019).

show ever, came under the spotlight when adverts for cosmetic surgery aired during the breaks. MYA Cosmetic Surgery's advert featured a group of gorgeous people lounging around in various luxury holiday condos. It's not to say there's anything wrong with cosmetic surgery, but there was widespread uproar about MYA's cynicism, to imply that a Love Island body was just one surgical procedure away. Ultimately the Advertising Standards Agency (ASA) banned them, saying that they were 'harmful' and 'irre-sponsible'. But it wasn't just the adverts that left people feeling bad about themselves:

> Seeing the girls bodies on love island literally makes me want to starve myself
>> – Livvy Mcalpine (@LivvyMcalpine) June 5, 2018

> All these girls bodies are making me never want to eat again #LoveIsland
>> – B (@bethanyellennx) June 4, 2018

By tracking the body shape of decades' worth of Miss America's contestants, researchers from the University of Missouri-Kansas City have shown that the new feminine ideal is no longer just thin, it is thin *and* toned. The waif look is out, big butts and tiny waists are in, but these physical ideals are just as hard to attain. The principles of #fitnotthin and #strongnotskinny are supposed to be founded on resistance to impossible beauty standards but they make people feel just as rubbish. Research shows that 'fitspiration' trends on Instagram leads to negative mood, body dissatisfac-tion and decreased self-esteem.[12] #Fitspiration is a new form of Puritanism – it signals those personal qualities which are prized

---

12 www.ncbi.nlm.nih.gov/pubmed/26176993 and www.ncbi.nlm.nih.gov/pubmed/25528369.

above all others: self control, discipline, productivity, wealth and a life long commitment to work.

Get shredded in six weeks!

To say that men are unencumbered by issues of body esteem would be patently untrue. It's well documented that cosmetic plastic surgery rates have soared in recent years, but by far the main reason for this is the number of men now going under the knife. Where eating disorders are typically associated with young girls and women, the number of adult men being admitted to hospital with an eating disorder has skyrocketed by 70 per cent over the past six years.[13]

In the same way that feminine beauty ideals reflect the values of the time, it is also true of masculine ideals. Today, an 'ideal' male body shape is not a million miles from the statues of Ancient Greece or ripped torsos of Renaissance paintings, but bulging muscles haven't always been an indicator of masculinity. In fact, throughout most of Europe's recent past, physical might was considered coarse and vulgar. Muscles were reserved for the labouring classes who spent their days working on the land. It was the enviable sedentary lifestyles of the upper classes, and their slim frames, that were the marker of class and privilege.

Beauty ideals remind us who holds power and who sets the agenda. Today's beauty standards expose just how uncomfortable our society is with 'non-normative' bodies: with gender queer bodies, disabled bodies and all other kinds of bodies that do not fit into the imagined ideal. Power is hitting the gym for two hours a day. It's being able to spend a fortune on health and beauty products that are inaccessible for the vast majority of working people.

---

13 www.theguardian.com/society/2017/jul/31/eating-disorders-in-men-rise-by-70-in-nhs-figures (last accessed 01/2019).

Areas of the media are responding at last to demands for greater representation. But whether or not this will challenge the root causes of why there is inequality in the first place is still hotly debated. For some, getting the right bodies in front of the camera and in the media is an end in itself. For others, just focussing on representation will never be enough. For instance, while we're increasingly seeing greater representation of people of colour in the media we consume, we've also witnessed a huge spike in the number of hate crimes in the West. In the US, there has been a nearly 23 per cent increase in religion-based hate crimes over the years 2017 and 2018 and a 37 per cent spike in anti-Jewish hate crimes.[14] In the UK, the number of recorded hate crimes has more than doubled over the years 2013 to 2018.[15]

Beauty standards (however impossible) tell us a lot about the values and histories of a society. So, they are not going anywhere. Nonetheless, as Kush, Naomi and Saff have all articulated above, there is solace in thinking critically about what society deems beautiful, and which bodies are valued and which are not. In the words of 18-year-old Simrun:

Simrun, 18

Ideals of beauty change around the world. In India, where my family are from, having a full nose and curves is the ultimate ideal beauty. Having a big nose means you have a strong character. Having curves means you're well fed and nourished. However, it's very different in the Western world. We have to appreciate what your background is. If you come from a different country, you may not fit the beauty ideal. I found this

---

14   www.theguardian.com/us-news/2018/nov/13/fbi-data-hate-crimes-rise-us-report.

15   https://assets.publishing.service.gov.uk/government/uploads/system/uploads/attachment_data/file/748598/hate-crime-1718-hosb2018.pdf.

very tough in school – because when guys went for girls it was a very specific type and as an ethnic minority, my type wasn't usually chosen. But as you get older you realise that these are other people's ideals, not yours. I think that if you are healthy, there's nothing to worry about. People come in all different shapes and sizes: I think everyone is beautiful.

Chapter 5

Sexual consent: No means no

Between 1975 and 1980, Peter Sutcliffe murdered 13 women and attempted to kill seven others. Dubbed the 'Yorkshire Ripper', Sutcliffe claimed that the voice of God had instructed him to eradicate all sex workers. Much like his Victorian counterpart, the murdering spree sent ripples of fear up and down the country. The press pumped out daily stories about the killer, hurling accusations at men in the public eye and providing gory details about the Ripper's victims.

With the Ripper still at large, the local police force made an official statement, suggesting that all women should remain inside after dark. Little did they realise, but their cautionary advice would lead to the greatest mass mobilisation of British women in decades. In 1977, the first Reclaim the Night march was held in Leeds. Women took to the streets, pouring out of their homes in their thousands shouting, 'No curfew on women – curfew on men'.

It was a clear mandate: the fault of sexual violence does not lie on the shoulders of survivors. In the case of the Yorkshire Ripper, they said that the problem lay with a disturbed paranoid schizophrenic and a society that objectifies women. Women should not have to stay indoors. Their indignation came after a lifetime of being told that if you wear short skirts, if you drink too much or flirt with your boss then it is your responsibility – you opened the door to rape. Instead, the protesters shifted the focus away from victims, towards the perpetrator, by making this an issue of consent: 'Whatever we wear, wherever we go, yes means yes and no means no!'

The 1977 Reclaim the Night movement was adamant that dominant attitudes towards sexual violence had to be addressed. Forty years later, how much has changed?

The law

The Sexual Offences Act 2003 for England and Wales says that a person consents to something if they 'agree by choice and have the freedom and capacity to make that choice'. In relation to sex, this means they are capable of saying yes to penetration, touching or any other sexual activity. The words 'freely' and 'actively' are key here. The law says that if someone is:

- Asleep
- Under the influence of drugs or alcohol
- Under the age of consent, 16 in the UK
- Coerced
- Manipulated
- Intentionally misled

Then it is non-consensual sex, in other words rape or assault.

The maximum sentence for sexual violence might be life imprisonment, but in practice it rarely plays out like that. The vast majority of sexual violence cases never even see the courts. 15 per cent of survivors in the UK report their rape to the authorities. Of that 15 per cent, only 5.7 per cent lead to a conviction.[1] These

---

1   www.independent.co.uk/news/uk/crime/rape-women-reporting-police-disclosure-evidence-phone-victims-commissioner-a8483411.html (last accessed 01/2019).

figures are even more startling when you consider that in the UK, the total number of rapes has almost doubled since 2013–14.[2] As the #MeToo movement highlighted, sexual violence is endemic, but the legal system has catastrophically failed to protect people.

There are differences of opinion about why the law falls short and what can be improved. For instance, with 90 per cent of sexual violence cases happening between people that know each other, some have shown that the justice system fails to accommodate the difficulty of bringing the law into relationships.[3] Others have pointed to public sector cuts, and the fact that there are simply not enough domestic violence services. But there is also a fundamental reason that gets to the heart of the inequalities within a justice system that treats some people as more worthy of listening to than others.

'Laws are like spiders' webs'

At the age of 19, Brock Turner was in a position many would kill for. He was an exceptionally brilliant athlete at one of the top universities in the world; he was a three-time All-American swimmer; and had realisable dreams of joining the US Olympic swimming team after graduation.

On 15 January 2015, two Swedish students discovered Turner lying on an intoxicated and unconscious 22-year-old woman behind a large dustbin on his campus grounds. The students, realising that something was wrong, approached Turner. When he saw them coming, Turner tried to run away, but they restrained him and called the police.

---

2   www.ons.gov.uk/peoplepopulationandcommunity/crimeandjustice/articles/
sexualoffencesinenglandandwales/yearendingmarch2017#sexual-offences-
recorded-by-the-police.

3   https://rapecrisis.org.uk/statistics.php.

Turner's trial kick-started an international conversation about consent and sexual violence. During his defence, Turner claimed that after a night of kissing and dancing at a university fraternity party, he and 'Emily Doe' (not her real name) had agreed to go back to his place. He said that on the way home, they had simply tripped and fallen.

Emily's account did not corroborate his. Emily had regained consciousness at around 4 a.m., remembering very little of the evening. However, she was adamant that she didn't consent to anything with Turner. Her sister confirmed this – she recalled Turner making multiple attempts to kiss Emily, but that she had repeatedly pulled away. Her assertion that it was not consensual, that she was assaulted was backed up by the hospital staff in the courtroom, who confirmed that she had experienced 'significant trauma' (physical injury or bruising) including 'penetrating trauma', resulting from the attack.

The courts ultimately found Turner guilty. He was convicted of three counts of assault, including attempted rape, and faced a maximum period of fourteen years in jail. In the judge's sentencing, it was decided that he should face much shorter time because (in the words of the judge) a longer period would have a 'severe impact' on Turner and his aspiring career as an Olympic swimmer. In the end, he was only sentenced to six months, of which he served three.

There was international outrage. Not only was it argued that men's careers are not always ruined by allegations of sexual assault – Johnny Depp and Donald Trump being among those that emerged unscathed after ample accusations – but that in the eyes of the law, and society at large, some people are believed and others not.

The prison system is institutionally rife with its own problems – not least, racism and classism – and simply throwing perpetrators behind bars will bring up a whole host of additional problematic consequences. Sexual violence is the consequence of misogyny and leaning on the penal system to tackle crime doesn't get to the root cause of why misogyny and gender-based violence exists in the first place. It has to be asked who the law protects and who it serves. It's easy to jail a black teenager for petty drug crime, but a lot harder to prosecute a rich white CEO who has been repeatedly harassing his employees. It tells us something that Greek political philosopher Anarchasis knew when he wrote in the sixth century BCE, well over 2,000 years ago: 'Written laws are like spiders' webs; they will catch, it is true, the weak and poor, but would be torn in pieces by the rich and powerful.'[4]

After Turner's sentencing, Emily wrote a statement, detailing what happened to her. It was an online viral sensation, having now been read well over eleven million times and counting, making it what can only be described as a precursor of the #MeToo movement. Here, she's recounting the prosecution's interrogation of her in the trial:

> Did you drink in college? You said you were a party animal? How many times did you blackout? Did you party at frats? Are you serious with your boyfriend? Are you sexually active with him? When did you start dating? Would you ever cheat? Do you have a history of cheating? What do you mean when you said you wanted to reward him? Do you remember what time you woke up? Were you wearing your cardigan? What colour was your cardigan? Do you remember any more from that night? No? Okay, we'll let Brock fill it in.

Emily was cornered and undermined over and over by the prosecution. It was said that she was lying and unhinged, that she was an unfaithful alcoholic – and that because she was so drunk, she was complicit. While Turner has the privilege to be innocent until

---

4   Plutarch, *Parallel Lives*, 'Solon' Book 5, Section 2.

proven guilty, Emily is subjected to the reverse: she was already presumed guilty.

There are, of course, some cases where rape is fabricated. However, in the UK, the number of cases that are considered untrue by the courts is put between two to eight per cent, almost exactly the same proportion as any other criminal accusation, like theft or fraud.[5] And of these cases, the reason that the majority of them fall through is because there's not enough evidence, and not because it was made it up. Yet, although 'cry-rape' is grossly exaggerated there remains a pervasive culture of not believing survivors.

Professor Kate Manne, author of best-selling *Down Girl: The Logic of Misogyny* calls this phenomenon 'himpathy', the disproportionate sympathy that powerful men enjoy when they are involved in cases of sexual violence, intimate partner violence or any other kind of misogynistic act.[6] She shows that in these cases society leaps to protect the male perpetrator, whether that's expressing concern about the damage to his future, to excusing him for 'just a mistake' or more generally to the energy spent massaging his ego and pouring care, respect and nurture onto him. His wellbeing is prioritised above and beyond everyone else. Manne argues that what makes himpathy so hard to challenge is that there is the pro-social morality bound up with the emotion of sympathy: 'Sympathy and empathy are pro-social moral emotions, which makes it especially hard to convince people that when they skew toward the powerful and against the vulnerable, they become a source of systemic injustice'.[7] The Brock Turner case is not an extreme case; once you spot it – himpathy is everywhere.

---

5   http://kunskapsbanken.nck.uu.se/nckkb/nck/publik/fil/visa/197/different.

6   Kate Manne, *Down Girl: The Logic of Misogyny* (London: Penguin, 2019).

7   www.nytimes.com/2018/09/26/opinion/brett-kavanaugh-hearing-himpathy.html (last accessed 12/2018).

The grey area

Sex is not a legal contract, and consent can be messy. The slogan 'No means No' is fundamental, but by implying that consent is always so simple, it fails to get to the heart of the messy tangle of human emotions involved. In Turner's case, consent was not given and force was used – it's a clear case of non-consensual sexual assault. However, there are many other instances where it becomes harder to see consent in terms of a binary yes and no. For instance, someone can say yes and then change their mind. Or say yes but feel pressured into making that decision. It might even be someone that you love and desire putting that pressure on you, confusing the idea of consent. Ideally, consent would be an enthusiastic 'YES', but so often consent is not conveyed like that.

Joe, 17

The most common non-consensual situation is when you're drunk. When two people are drunk, is it even possible to give consent? Bad situations happen all the time at our age. This is when teenage girls and boys are experimenting with drugs and drink. Guys will get drunk and then wake up in the morning, not remember what they did and feel really bad about it.

Clearly, consent is incredibly complicated, but that doesn't mean it should be ignored. Turner built his defence around the claim that Emily did actually agree to go home with him, but that she was too drunk to remember. This murky area of consent is found in statements that are all too common:

- We were both completely wasted, sure, but we were both obviously up for it
- We're in a relationship so we can have sex all the time!

- Well, he didn't say no . . .
- She was wearing a really short skirt: she was obviously up for it
- What was he expecting if he went upstairs to bed with her?
- I didn't know she was asleep

In some instances, people experience the 'freeze-response', where they are unable to say no because of fear, shame or any other emotion. The very fact that it is complicated means it requires greater attention and more willingness to give consent. The majority of people know when their consent has been compromised, whether that's at the start or along the way during a sexual encounter. But in a society where lack of clarity around consent is common sense, rape can be excused by others as an accident – merely a misunderstanding. This is where rape culture comes into play.

Blurred lines

After a tragic incident, a beautiful young woman ends up in a coma. Years pass by, until her devastated family are left with no option but to presume she will never recover. They are eventually granted permission to take her home, where she remains, sleeping for years until a young man hears about her beauty and decides that he wants to marry her. Determined that she must he his, he hatches a plan. He finds out where she lives and breaks into her house in the middle of the night. Once he's safely inside, he climbs the stairs to her bedroom, where he finds her lying unconscious. Upon seeing her, love and admiration overwhelm him. Prince Charming moves towards the bed, leans over Sleeping Beauty and kisses her passionately.

Woven into the fabric of the myths and stories that build Western culture are ideas about the ultimate expression of love. Sleeping Beauty is just one example where non-consent is venerated and men pursuing women is game and normal. These narratives around non-consent are ever present today.

> OK, now he was close
> Tried to domesticate you
> But you're an animal
> Baby, it's in your nature
> Just let me liberate you
> You don't need no papers
> That man is not your mate
> And that's why I'm gon' take you

> [...]

> I'll give you something big enough to tear your ass in two

> [...]

> I hate these blurred lines!
> I know you want it
> I know you want it
> I know you want it

Feminists from the 1970s coined the term 'Rape Culture' to describe the kind of society where non-consent is considered normal and fine. They argued that when we look at cultural outputs – film, music, TV, etc – there's a pervasive tolerance for non-consent. Not only is heterosexuality considered the de facto sexuality, but there's a romantic script which states that man pursues woman, woman resists and then woman succumbs. 'Blurred Lines' was controversial, but it was just a more explicit admission of what we see everywhere else, from James Bond, to *Twilight* to *Friends*. In the end 'Blurred Lines' made well over $17 million and both Robin Thicke and Pharrell walked away with $5 million each. It raises the thorny question about how we should treat the work of successful artists who have been accused of sexual violence, or make light of sexual violence – Woody Allen and Harvey Weinstein included – but donating the profits to survivors of domestic violence would be a start.

Recognising the significance of rape culture is essential, because it's reflected in people's attitudes towards sex and consent. If you were chatting someone up and they physically pushed you away, would you consider that a sign to stop? The majority of young adults wouldn't think so. In a study of over 1,000 18–25 year-olds, over half did not think that someone physically pushing them away means no. The same study showed that 60 per cent of young people would not read someone crying during sex as non-consent; and that more than one in five people expect intercourse after other kinds of touching. #Metoo was a global expression of something many of us have known for a long time: that respect for consent is rare and non-consent is common.

The cost of pleasure

S, 20

Well this happened just recently. I had been with my boyfriend for a few months and he had just got back from a long holiday. I really wasn't in the mood but I wanted him to feel desired, to feel loved and to feel good. So I consented to having sex with him that night. The next morning I felt terrible. I couldn't stop crying. Everything hurt.

In the midst of the MeToo movement, an article from *The Week* magazine titled 'The Female Price of Male Pleasure' went viral. It spoke about those sexual encounters that sit badly, just like S's, but isn't necessarily about rape. In the piece, she argues that this kind of experience is actually the norm. Research shows that 30 per cent of cis-women report pain during heterosexual vaginal sex, 72 per cent report pain during anal sex, and 'large proportions' don't tell their partners when sex hurts.[8] Why would someone endure something that is not only unpleasant, but actually painful? This is the everyday, lived reality of living under a system of such inequality; the crushing weight of pressure to conform to someone else's pleasure at the expense of your own.

It can be hard to say no. Historically, women have performed the vast majority of caring roles in the economy and this dynamic manifests in the most minute interpersonal exchanges. By no means is it only women who are vulnerable to this kind of power imbalance. As we will see in Chapter 8 on sexual violence, there's a direct relationship between who has economic and political power in society and who is less vulnerable to sexual violence or forms of gender based violence. LGBTQ people, for instance, are statistically more likely to be survivors, and women of colour are more likely than white women to be subjected to gender-based violence. As Harry, aged 17, explains, the scale of sexual violence is staggering.

Harry, 17

One thing that the #MeToo movement revealed is the amount of women who have been through some kind of unwarranted sexual advances. I spoke to my mum about this, she reckons that every woman will experience something. Not rape necessarily, but some kind of sexual misconduct. Every woman will experience this at some point in their lives. The statistics prove how bad it is.

---

8   www.ncbi.nlm.nih.gov/pubmed/25648245.

When I hear about this I feel very upset. I think most young boys must also feel like this. Because sometimes you see someone on the street and you think they're quite good looking, you think okay . . . But then if this many women have gone through this then what am I capable of? And what are the boys around me capable of? I've never done anything or thought of anything but it's just like – Jesus Christ . . .

Where now?

The BDSM (Bondage, Discipline, Submission and Sadomasochism) community was thrust into the public consciousness after the sex life of Mr Grey became raunchy reading material for the world. Despite being the fifth best-selling book of all time, we can learn more from BDSM than *Fifty Shades of Grey* author E. L. James would have imagined.

While BDSM is a catchall term that involves a number of different erotic practices, the central tenet is that participants take on unequal roles. Ranging from physical restraint, whipping to erotic humiliation, the terms 'top'/ 'sub' (submissive) and 'bottom'/'dom' (dominant) are used to describe these different power dynamics. It goes without saying that if you're going to engage in knife or wax play, there are obvious health and safety warnings attached. It is therefore unsurprising that consent has always been a cornerstone of kink.

Some in the BDSM community use a Yes, No, Maybe chart. Every sexual act you can think of is written down and then categorised into: what you would like to do/would enjoy doing, things you might consider and then those that you would never dream of trying. Your partner also fills out the list, and then the conversation begins: what do you have in common? What would you negotiate and what would you absolutely never do? And then the conversation happens again. Each act, each time is – ideally –

driven by a commitment to consent. Not everyone will want to try out tickle torture, and it may not be practical to print out this kind of chart for every encounter, but given how pervasive non-consent is, it is not such a stretch to give the same level of attention to all kinds of sex. Forty years later and the rallying cry of 'No Means No' still holds true.

Chapter 6

Contraceptives: 'If you have sex you will get pregnant and die'

Humans have gone to the end of the world to prevent pregnancy. At some point beaver testicles, crocodile dung, earwax, cat bones, spider carcasses, honey, bleach and poisonous herbs have all played their part. Hippocrates, the Greek physician and 'Father of Medicine' recommended drinking copper to keep fertility levels down. The notorious lover, Casanova, wrote in his journal that he encouraged his partners to insert half a lemon into their vaginas as a spermicide. None of these methods are recommended (although Casanova, it turns out, was right – lemon does indeed have mild spermicidal effects).

Preventing pregnancy is not the only use for contraceptives. For many, they are a lifeline: a way to treat medical conditions, to maintain sexual health and to have multiple partners without worry. In spite of assumptions, and the way that heterosexuality is taught as the default sexuality in schools, contraceptives are not exclusively used by straight and cis people. Trans and queer people also get pregnant, and everyone – regardless of sexuality – is vulnerable to infection. In the words of queer, non-binary activist Sebastian Zulch, 'being gay isn't a Get Out of Jail Free Card – STDs don't discriminate'.[1]

---

1   http://helloflo.com/the-problem-with-associating-contraceptives-with-only-straight-penetrative-sex/.

Contraceptives are for all and they have shaped human history. Where lumps of wood and beaver testicles were once thought of as preferable to pregnancy, the options today are on the whole less painful and easier to come by. In the UK there are 15 methods of contraception and pregnancy prevention available. However, I will focus on the four most commonly used here – condoms, the pill, abortion and natural planning.

Condoms

Condoms have been around for thousands of years. Unlike today's latex, some of the earliest condoms were made of silk paper, very thin hollow horns and animal intestines. Today, between six to nine billion condoms are sold every year and while there are few intestines in sight, condoms can be ribbed, vegan, extra small, extra large, spray-on and even 'smart', measuring sexual performance and calories burned among other things. While the condom's form has changed, one thing has remained constant: wherever condoms go, controversy is never far behind.

Young people tend to be seen as the arch-culprits of not practicing safe sex but the older generations are just as guilty. In the UK today, STI rates among the over 60s are booming. In what is being referred to as 'a crisis', an NHS campaign was launched in early 2019 to give out free condoms to frisky pensioners in an attempt to quell the rise. Among younger generations, STI rates are also on the up, with around one young person being diagnosed with an infection every four minutes in England. Worryingly, the number of adolescents living with HIV also rose by a third between 2005 and 2016.[2]

As we'll see throughout this chapter, not everyone demands the same thing from contraception. In the words of Saff E. D., a 21-year-old student:

---

2 www.avert.org/professionals/hiv-social-issues/key-affected-populations/young-people.

> I am Muslim and I never had a religious sex education. In the Muslim community there is a huge stigma around sex. I don't want children, and throughout most of my childhood I thought that Muslims couldn't use birth control – so my only solution was to say that I was never ever going to get married. I had to Google 'are Muslims allowed to use birth control', which of course we are, but it's worrying that that was an actual question I had and I had to turn to Google for that. I think schools should tailor their sex ed for their students based on what they need.

There are religious considerations when it comes to contraceptives, but there are also important differences relating to sexuality and sexual practice. As Nicky Ryan from Free 2B, a South London organisation that supports LGBTQ+ young people, explained:

> Contraception is always looked at from a heteronormative point of view. Even when I go to the doctor, they always say what are you doing about contraception. That's when they say, 'is your husband wearing a condom?' I'm like, I've been telling you for years that I'm with a woman. I'm a confident person I can tell the doctor how it is. But it's extremely extremely frustrating. I can't tell you how frustrating it is. For young people it's probably even worse. Sexual health clinics still have a lot of work to do.

As Nicky points out, within the NHS – just like the rest of society – there remains the widespread assumption that everyone is straight. Stonewall's 2017 'Unhealthy Attitudes' report revealed that LGBTQ+ people face discrimination and a lack of understanding when accessing health services. Even though healthcare providers have a legal duty under the Equalities Act of 2010 to treat LGBTQ+ people fairly and without discrimination, this doesn't match up to people's experiences, Nicky included.

Due to being afraid of discrimination from medical practitioners, the following proportion of LGBTQ+ people have avoided some kind of medical treatment or attention:

- One in seven LGBTQ+ people have avoided treatment
- Almost two in five trans people and a third of non-binary people have avoided treatment
- One in four LGBTQ+ people aged 18–24 have avoided treatment
- One in five LGBTQ+ disabled people have avoided treatment
- One in five PoC LGBTQ+ people have avoided treatment[3]

In the UK, lesbian and bisexual women are twice as likely to have never had a cervical smear test.[4] Gay men are far more likely to catch an STI, but one in four gay and bisexual men in the UK have never been tested at all.[5]

The NHS was one of the first health systems in the world to provide free contraception and free treatment for STDs, but sexual health clinics today have either been closed down or are struggling to survive. Much like the rest of the NHS, they have been 'cut to the bone' by budget funding cuts.[6] Nurses report that patients are turned away every day, with one doctor at a hospital in South London saying that around 300 people every week are left untreated. As Nicky Ryan says, sexual health clinics have a long way to go to be more inclusive – and a lot of work is going on already – but when they're battling for survival, this important work will invariably remain neglected.

3   Chaka L. Bachmann and Becca Gooch, *LGBT in Britain, Health Report* (Stonewall, 2017), 13–14.

4   www.stonewall.org.uk/sites/default/files/stonewall-guide-for-the-nhs-web.pdf.

5   www.stonewall.org.uk/sites/default/files/stonewall-guide-for-the-nhs-web.pdf.

6   www.theguardian.com/society/2018/dec/30/sexual-disease-gonorrhoea-health-cuts-local-authority-sexually-transmitted.

The pill

Women are 'needed to bring about the increase of the human race. Whatever their weaknesses, women possess one virtue that cancels them all: they have a womb and they can give birth' – Martin Luther, father of the Protestant Church

The significance of the birth control pill has not gone unnoticed. When it hit its fiftieth anniversary, *TIME* magazine said the pill had 'rearranged the furniture of human relations'.[7] In 1969, Ashley Montagu, a British-American Anthropologist went so far to claim that 'the pill ranks in importance with the discovery of fire', that the technology had already upturned 'age-old beliefs, practices and institutions'.[8] Today 3.5 million people in Britain and approximately 100 million around the world use it, and the number continues to rise. But the path to where we are now has been thorny and in some cases, deadly.

The very first pill was pioneered by four individuals who joined forces under a shared vision: Margaret Sanger, Katherine McCormick, Gregory Pincus and John Rock. The gang of four were blinded by determination and enacted questionable politics to get what they wanted. Some of the pill's early supporters were hardened eugenicists, keen to see the improvement of the genetics of the human race. Sanger herself had originally thought about calling the pill 'race control' rather than 'birth control'. In her words: 'The world and almost all of our civilisation for the next 25 years is going to depend upon a simple, cheap, safe contraceptive to be used in poverty-stricken slums and jungles, and among the most ignorant people.'[9]

---

7 http://time.com/5405987/history-of-contraception/.
8 www.theguardian.com/books/2015/mar/18/the-birth-of-the-pill-jonathan-eig-review-sex-drugs-population-control. Accessed February 2019.
9 Lara V. Marks, *Sexual Chemistry: A History of the Contraceptive Pill* (New Haven: Yale University Press, 2001), 13.

Contraception in the 1930s and 1940s was illegal in most US states, but this wasn't the only reason they struggled to find and keep people in their experiment. A number of participants passed away and many others experienced extreme side effects, including mood change and bloating. The dropout rate became impossible to ignore and they decided to move their first large-scale trials to Puerto Rico, where regulation was looser and human life was considered cheaper. They also gave the pill to patients in a US women's mental asylum without their consent.

In time, the pill was ready to go on the market. Contraception was still illegal. So on 10 June 1957, the sale of 'Enovid' was approved in the US to help 'regulate the menstrual cycle' and was marketed as the 'miracle tablet'. On the back of the packet one side effect was listed as 'preventing ovulation'. Within two years, 1.2 million American people were using it. The first birth control pill was introduced by the NHS in 1961 by Enoch Powell, then Minister for Health, but only for married women. It wasn't until 1967 that single women were allowed a prescription, but in practice it was well into the early seventies that women in Britain and America were still pretending to be married, passing round battered wedding rings in waiting rooms just to get a packet.

The original pill, Enovid, contained over ten times the amount of hormones than in most contraceptive pills today, so it's no surprise that the health complications have significantly diminished since its early days. Despite its sinister history, the pill has been undeniably transformative. Not only does it manage fertility and regulate menstruation, but it's also used to treat acne and hormonal problems like PCOS and endometriosis. While in its short history the pill has been blamed for promiscuity and for destroying marriages, having the ability to choose whether or not to get pregnant has been liberating for immeasurable numbers of people. Some older women who witnessed the transformative effect of the pill have accused younger generations of taking the pill for granted. 'Young women don't realise what hell it was [before the arrival of the pill]' says the fashion designer Mary Quant. 'The perpetual anxiety. It was a real revolution.'[10]

At the start of 2019, it was announced that the seven-day break each month for 'pill-bleeding' was unnecessary; that it had been created to mimic the experience of menstruation, but that in reality the bleeding bears absolutely no resemblance to a real period. Many felt hoodwinked and disempowered that they had been taking medication for years without fully understanding the side effects. It left many asking what else we were not told about the pill.

The links between birth control and mental health problems are discussed among friends, but many doctors will assure you that the pill does not affect your mood. However, two recent and large-scale studies from the University of Copenhagen told a different story. They showed that the rise of a diagnosis of depression increases by 23 per cent for those who are on the combined pill.[11] For users of all hormonal contraception, the risk of suicide is threefold.[12] For teenagers, it's even more stark: the risk of clinical depression is a whopping 80 per cent higher for people taking hormonal contraception.

Open a contraceptive pill packet and you'll find over 100 listed side effects. Beyond the mental health complications there are also physical risks, such as weight gain, nausea, fertility issues, headaches, reduced libido and blood clots. Every single body is different, so it's natural that we'd all have different experiences with the medication. For many people the pill is Sanger's 'magic pill', but for many others it can take an enormous physical and mental toll.

---

10   www.theguardian.com/society/2010/jun/06/rachel-cooke-fifty-years-the-pill-oral-contraceptive.

11   https://jamanetwork.com/journals/jamapsychiatry/fullarticle/2552796.

12   https://ajp.psychiatryonline.org/doi/abs/10.1176/appi.ajp.2017.17060616?journalCode=ajp&.

It's impossible to ignore how disproportionately gendered this burden is. As soon as there were the first grumblings about a contraceptive pill for women, there were also attempts to develop a male version. But it wasn't until the early 1970s when the Chinese and US governments launched studies to find sperm-suppressing chemicals that real steps were taken to find a male pill. Chinese researchers ran a number of trials of a chemical called gossypol, a derivative of cotton plants. However, while these pills did reduce sperm count, a number of those involved never got back to their original fertility levels.[13]

The quest to make a 'male contraceptive pill' has been unsuccessful, grossly underfunded and thwarted. The main reason most research has been cut short is because of the 'severe side effects' participants recorded. In 2016 one of the most extensive male contraceptive trials launched in ten sites around the world with support from the UN and World Health Organisation. It had astonishingly successful results in 96 per cent of the participants (2016). However, an independent panel argued that the pill was unsafe to be released to the public because of the 'severe' side effects. What did they include? Among others: acne, general mood and libido changes.[14] Sound familiar?

Abortion

After decades of campaigning, May 2018 saw the Irish people vote by a landslide to repeal the Eighth Amendment, a law that prohibited abortion in nearly all circumstances.

Abortion might have been illegal over all those years, but procedures still look place. Every year 2,000 women took illegal and unsafe pills to terminate pregnancy and eleven women

---

13   http://time.com/longform/male-pill/.

14   http://press.endocrine.org/doi/10.1210/jc.2016-2141?url_ver=Z39.88-2003& rfr_id=ori%3Arid%3Acrossref.org&rfr_dat=cr_pub%3Dpubmed&.

travelled to mainland Britain every day to have an abortion, or be authorised by a clinician to take abortive medicines at home. Behind each statistic is a story. Some were survivors of rape or abuse, but others simply didn't want to have a child.

Anti-abortion laws were at the heart of the most fundamental governing principles of the Irish nation. They were introduced in 1983, during a time when the Catholic Church and the Vatican were concerned about developments such as Roe vs. Wade and the legalisation of abortion around Europe. Ireland was held up as an example to the world where you could put anti-choice laws right into the beating heart of a nation's identity.

The results of the 2018 referendum are seismic. More than 66 per cent of the Irish population gave a resounding 'yes' to repeal the Eighth Amendment. Ireland was the most recent country to make steps to legalise abortion, but there are still 26 countries around the world where it is illegal. There are also 37 other countries where abortion is only permitted when it's necessary to save the life of the mother, and a further 36 countries restrict access unless an abortion is necessary to protect a mothers health.[15]

In the UK, one in three cis-women will have an abortion at some point in their lives. But what is the law surrounding it? Prior to the Abortion Act of 1967 in the UK, anyone seeking a termination would have to go before a committee and explain why they needed an abortion. Today, there are still limitations. Two doctors have to confirm that they meet the criteria laid out in the 1967 Abortion Act, including that 'the termination is necessary to prevent grave permanent injury to the physical or mental health of the pregnant woman'. While there is a lot of progress, 'because I don't want to be pregnant' or 'there are other things I'd rather do with my life' isn't enough. Pro-choice campaigners say that it's essential that people are given a decision to decide how their future will be. At many points in our lives, pregnancy is not possible or not preferred.

---

15   www.guttmacher.org/report/abortion-worldwide-2017.

Aashni, 17

A lot of girls at my school have already got kids and the rest have a boyfriend and want to have a baby. Sometimes I do get baby fever, but it's not simple. Firstly if you're brown and he's brown your parents are going to kill you. Secondly, you're so young! How you going to afford it? Obviously if you have a kid your life isn't ending, but I want to go university and get a job. I feel like it's a trend, getting pregnant. It's a proper trend. People just don't realise how hard it can be.

Anti-choice campaigners argue that legalising abortion will open the floodgates and encourage people to use abortion as a primary contraceptive. But there is no evidence that this happens: the difference in abortion rates between countries where it is legal and illegal is practically immaterial.[16] As Ireland shows so clearly, even when abortions are illegal, people will still find ways to terminate their pregnancies. What's at stake here is safety, and giving people choice over their own body, away from shame and stigma.

Back to the future

One of the oldest forms of pregnancy prevention, the 'Catholic technique' as it is sometimes called, has resurfaced. Concerned about the potential side effects of hormonal birth control, many are turning to the past and looking at technology for answers. There are now apps such as Natural Cycles, the 'world's first contraceptive app', which allows people to plan sex around their menstruation cycle. The company's claim was that after inputting data about your cycle, they could provide the most accurate,

---

16 www.guttmacher.org/news-release/2018/new-report-highlights-worldwide-variations-abortion-incidence-and-safety.

bespoke account of your fertility levels. On the green days, go ahead, on red days – proceed with caution.

Within months, close to a million people around the world signed up to Natural Cycles. No more bloating, no more acne, mood changes and weight gain. But then the unwanted pregnancies started to happen. It turned out that Natural Cycles was not as 'highly accurate' as it claimed to be at all. In one month in a hospital in Stockholm, 37 women were reported to have come in for an abortion having used Natural Cycles as contraception.

In spite of attempts around the world to crack down on reproductive rights, there is every reason to imagine that the future is bright. The popularity of Natural Cycles tells us many are unhappy with the current state of play and that huge investment is being pumped into alternatives. Technology to track fertility levels – or 'Femtech' – is expected to be a 50 billion-dollar industry by 2025 and there are already developments to create a more accurate and effective version of Natural Cycles. With enough investment and – importantly – with the right political motivations, there's every possibility that give it 100 years and it's possible that the pill and implant will be seen as outdated as anything the Ancient Romans were using thousands of years ago.

Chapter 7

Virginity: Purity

> Edward: This is unbearable. So many things I've wanted to give you – and this is what you decide to demand? Do you have any idea how painful it is, trying to refuse you, when you plead with me this way?
>
> Bella: Give me one good reason why tonight is not as good as any other night.
>
> – *Twilight* Meyer, *Eclipse*.[1]

Dreamy heartthrob Edward Cullen had been a virgin for hundreds and hundreds of years before he met Bella Swan at a high school in Forks, Washington. The pair immediately fall for each other. After longing stares over the school's canteen, after he saves her life – twice – and after Edward breaks into her father's house to watch her sleep, they declare their burning desire for one another. In line with committed Mormon and *Twilight* author Stephenie's sexual politics, Edward insists they wait until their wedding night. Much to the frustration of *Twilight*'s 100 million readers around the world, that would be a whole four books later.

The Bella-Edward trend is spreading. A 2018 report revealed that more than one in eight young people in the UK have not had sex before the age of twenty-six, making us a generation of the oldest virgins on record.[2] The UK is not alone. Every country

---

1 Stephenie Meyer, *Eclipse* (New York: Little, Brown and Company, 2006), 448.

2 www.telegraph.co.uk/news/2018/05/06/millennials-turned-sex-study-suggests-one-eight-still-virgins/.

where similar studies have been conducted show exactly the same trend. In Japan the numbers are at their most stark, with almost half of all people entering into their thirties not having had any sexual experience, at all.[3] The Japanese media are calling this *sekkusu shinai shokogun,* meaning 'celibacy syndrome', and have identified it as a national crisis, with some fearing that combined with an already stagnating population, Japan 'might eventually perish into extinction'.[4]

So what's going on? Birth control is largely available; if hook-ups are your thing, Tinder and Grinder make it available with a swipe; shaming words like 'perverted' have become 'kinky' and we are living through a time of hard-fought wins for LGBTQ+ people. However – and this will be music to some parents' ears – the figures are clear, young people are launching their sex lives much later. There's an abundance of theories attempting to explain why – ranging from anxiety disorders; helicopter parents; anti-depressants; fear of intimacy; careerism; smartphones; masturbation; pornography; sleep deprivation; economic crises and dating apps. But in short – we don't really know.

It's clear from the catastrophising headlines that the majority of the discourse around is not led by the experiences of young people. 'GENERATION VIRGIN: Millennials shun sex';[5] 'No sex please, we're millennials';[6] 'No sex, please, we're only 26: millennials cling to virginity'[7] and 'Millennials are too nervous to have

3   www.independent.co.uk/news/world/asia/japan-sex-problem-demographic-time-bomb-birth-rates-sex-robots-fertility-crisis-virgins-romance-porn-a7831041.html (last accessed 3/10/2018.

4   www.theguardian.com/world/2013/oct/20/young-people-japan-stopped-having-sex (last accessed 03/12/2018).

5   www.thesun.co.uk/news/6223123/millennials-shun-sex-as-one-in-eight-26-year-olds-reveal-they-are-virgins/.

6   www.dailymail.co.uk/news/article-5696417/Virgin-numbers-rise-UK-fear-intimacy.html.

7   www.thetimes.co.uk/edition/news/no-sex-please-were-only-26-millennials-cling-to-virginity-t9gxo3r6x.

sex.'[8] In this chapter, we'll look back at the cultural history of virginity, to understand what it actually means to be a virgin, and how that might impact many millions of young people around the world today who are either waiting or have decided that sex isn't for them.

Tainted love

Twilight might be the best-selling romance of our time, but back in 1200 it was *Floris and Blancheflour*, a French epic that took England by storm. With its magical twists and fantastical beasts, the love story dealt with epic themes of war, love, sacrifice and – just like *Twilight* – the big V. In the scene below, the rich King of Babylon is hunting for a new wife and is faced with a group of hopeful maidens. Overwhelmed by choice, the King calls upon the help of a magical fountain to aid his decision:

If any woman approaches [the fountain] who has slept with a
    man
And she kneels on the ground
To wash her hands,
The water will scream as though it were mad,
And turn as red as blood.
Whichever maiden causes the water to act thus
Shall soon be put to death.

And those that are clean maidens [virgins],
They may wash themselves in the stream.
The water will run silent and clear
It will not cause them any harm

---

8   www.thetimes.co.uk/article/millennials-too-nervous-to-have-sex-dg9kr9065.

This small section tells us three essential things about the traditional understanding of virginity. Firstly, that virginity is a dichotomy: either you are a virgin, or you are not. Secondly that virginity produces a physical transformation, and that this change is permanent and possible to detect. And finally, that virginity is a pure state of being reserved exclusively for women. *Floris* was written over 800 years ago, but the similarities between then and now are startling.

Either a Virgin or Not

The King's fountain has the magical ability to tell whether the maidens are virgins or not. On first appearances, the question 'are you a virgin?' might seem clear – but it's not so simple. What it means to lose your virginity will differ from person to person based on what your idea of sex is. In religious and cis-heterosexual traditions, it tends to be seen as the first time a person has penetrative sex. But what about non-heteronormative sexual practice?

In the words of Hanne Blank in her bestselling book *Virgin,* 'We live in a culture that does not appreciate ambiguity when it comes to either sexuality or morality, after all, and virginity is inextricably twined with both.'[9] However, this hasn't always been the case.

In Ancient Greek writing, for instance, it was sometimes understood as a characteristic – physical or abstract – but it was also described like an object, being seized (*lambanein*), an object that is owed respect (*terein*) or as an object or thing that has to be unwrapped (*lyein*). Thomas Aquinas, the thirteenth-century theologian, believed that virginity was a personal quality of temperance and 'chastity'. Chastity, for Aquinas wasn't just about sex, but it was also related to a kind of spiritual chastity that

9   Hanne Blank, *Virgin: The Untouched History* (London: Bloomberg Publishing, 2007).

rejected all things immoral. Within this definition, a simple yes or no would surely not suffice.

Virginity as a Physical Change

Floris tells us that virginity tests have a long history. The fountain being basically a fantastical apparatus created to determine whether or not a person is a virgin. Today, you will be unlikely to find a magic fountain, but nevertheless they persist. The majority of virginity tests would be a physical internal inspection of cis-women to check the state of her 'hymen', the membrane surrounding the vaginal opening.

The underlying principle – that penetrative sex breaks the hymen and causes irreversible change – reflects an outdated and inaccurate understanding of sex and gender. Not all cis-women are born with a hymen; not all cis-women have penetrative sex; not all women have female genitalia; *and* of the women that are born with a hymen and do have penetrative sex, it's extremely common for the hymen tissue to wear away during childhood and adolescence, through exercise or even menstruation.

Virginity tests come in different forms but they tend to have one thing in common: they serve to further control women's bodies and sexuality. During the Egyptian revolution in 2011, a group of female activists were rounded up by the police and subjected to forced virginity tests, or 'purity tests'. After initially denying that this had taken place, an Egyptian general was later found boasting about it to CNN: 'the girls who were detained are not like your daughter or mine. These girls who had camped out in tents with male protestors in Tahrir Square [in Cairo] [. . .] None of them were virgins'. These tests were delivered to strip away the political credibility of the activists who were, themselves, calling into question the legitimacy of the Egyptian state. As we've seen, there are no physical markers of virginity so the state's conclusions were redundant, but what they do tell us is important: that virginity is attached to a moral code.

Virginity and Purity

In the words of Hanne Blank 'virginity does not exist. It can't be weighed on a scale, sniffed out like a truffle or a smuggled bundle of cocaine, retrieved from the lost-and-found, or photographed for posterity [. . .] Virginity is as distinctively human a notion as philanthropy. We invented it. We developed it.'[10] Virginity might be relative; that doesn't mean it's irrelevant.

The word 'virgin' has gendered roots. It comes directly from the old French word *virgine*, meaning 'maiden', or a sexually inexperienced woman. In German the word for virgin is *jungfrau* meaning literally 'young women'. Much like the expectations of strength and power that are within the masculine ideal, sexual purity is an attribute of femininity that puts all kinds of women in a double bind. At its core, the fundamental assumption is that female sexuality is somehow tainted and impure. An example of the real life effect of these values is that where men might be called a stud or a player for having multiple partners, women can be called a slut or easy.

Just like the qualities of masculinity, having such unreachable aspirations for femininity creates a hierarchy of proximity. There are those at the top, who are most closely associated with moral purity, and then those that fall away from that ideal. This kind of hierarchy creates a divide between women: some are fallen, others angelic. Degrading images of women of colour in the media and porn, in particular, perpetuate the racist stereotype that gives white women access to sexual and moral purity alone. Women of colour are fetishised and sexualised, in different ways. Black women are represented as sexually dominant and wild in bed;

---

10   Blank, *Virgin: The Untouched History.*

Asian women as submissive and kinky; Latina women as feisty. We'll talk more about racial fetishisation in Chapter 10 on pornography, but it's significant to mention here that racism and misogyny have fed into the whore/angel distinction and that moral purity and innocence are only afforded to some women. As we'll see in Chapter 11, this kind of moralising has led to intense discrimination against sex workers.

Incel

Virginity means something different for men. The below case is clearly an extreme example of the pitfalls of the sexual expectations of masculinity, but it's still useful to draw out the logic.

On the evening of 23 May 2014, a 22-year-old man, Elliot Rodger, turned a gun on himself after a stabbing and shooting spree which left six people dead and fourteen injured. Rodger is now notorious, but not just because he joins the list of young American men who have killed their fellow students. Before he died, Rodger uploaded a biographical video and a link to his own autobiography, detailing why he believed he was compelled to take such a violent act.

The son of a wealthy British Hollywood producer, Rodger grew up in the English countryside before his family moved to an affluent neighbourhood of LA. All his life he knew privilege, but the other similarly wealthy children at his school bullied him repeatedly for years. His parents tried moving between schools but the taunting continued and he developed crippling social anxiety. His diary shows a maturing adolescent increasingly obsessed with getting rich and getting laid. His sense of injustice burns through the pages. In spite of maintaining that 'I am closest thing there is to a living God' Elliot was not popular with girls. He despised the boys who had girlfriends almost as much as the women who rejected him. He dropped out of school, gambled thousands and thousands of dollars, believing wealth would get him the girl of his dreams. When, of course, it didn't, resentment grew to rage. Rodger uploaded a stream of Vlogs. Describing himself as the 'ideal magnificent gentleman', he spits and hurls abuse at 'hot' girls and the 'chads' (men with girlfriends) that had got in his way – he railed and railed about his virginity. In the end, Rodger would call his murdering spree the 'Day of Retribution'. He said he had 'no choice but to enact revenge on the society' that 'denied' him sex.[11]

His autobiography has subsequently become something of a Bible for 'involuntary celibate' (or Incel) communities online, men who have had no sexual experiences and blame women for it. These fringe communities consider sex from women their right and Rodger a hero. Reddit and YouTube have tried to crack down on Incel videos and discussions, but like a game of cat and mouse, independent platforms spring up almost immediately. They all proudly talk about their hatred of women and chads and their respect for acts of violence against women.[12]

In April 2018, Alek Minassian killed ten people in Toronto, Canada. Moments before, he sent this tweet:

Private (recruit) Minassian Infantry 00010, wishing to speak to Sgt 4chan please. C23249161. The Incel Rebellion has already begun! We will overthrow all the Chads and Staceys! All hail the Supreme Gentleman Elliot Rodger!

The cases of Rodger and Minassian are the most extreme manifestations of male entitlement and misogyny. Clearly, not all men believe it is their right to own and have control over women's bodies, and thankfully not all men believe violence is just retribu-

---

11 https://medium.com/editorials-on-current-events/i-read-the-elliot-rodger-manifesto-so-you-dont-have-to-b0b66c629ca5.

12 www.newstatesman.com/science-tech/internet/2017/02/reddit-the-red-pill-interview-how-misogyny-spreads-online.

tion to women who deny them sex. However, it's an uncomfortable truth that their ideas about women are also reflected – to lesser degrees – in other places.

You could say that it's just a fairy tale, but the King of Babylon's magical fountain is extremely sexually violent. At the will of the King, the hopeful maidens who are found not to be virgins are immediately put to death – the King has total ownership over their bodies. With misogyny like this permeating culture for over 800 years, is it so surprising that this world produced Elliot Rodger?

Sex negative vs sex positive

Back to the millennial sex drought. Rather than moralising about failings of 'youth today', let's take another, sex positive, approach.

The term 'sex positive' is attributed to an Austrian psychoanalysis, Wilhelm Reich who proposed an alternative society to the 'sex negative' one that dominated twentieth-century Europe, which by and large taught that sex is shameful. The debate between sex negativity and positivity rose to prominence, however, in the 1970s during a major and irreparable ideological split within the women's movement, later called the 'Porn Wars', on whether or not pornography could be feminist. Sex negatives said no – that porn is a crude patriarchal tool that objectifies women's bodies. Sex positive feminists, however, disagreed, saying that sexual practice is up to the discretion of each person. They pointed out that the way many sex negative feminists talk about sex is remarkably similar to some of the most conservative strands of social values. Andrea Dworkin, for instance, argued that 'intercourse is the pure, sterile, formal expression of men's contempt for women.'[13]

It's fair to say that sex positivity dominates feminism today and has ricocheted out and away from activist groups, with kink and BDSM practically being household terms now. The focus of

---

13   Andrea Dworkin, *Intercourse* (New York: Basic Books 1987), 175.

sex positivity is to celebrate all forms of consensual sex and, in particular, to debunk the idea that some kinds of sex are morally right, and others wrong. It was made for types of sexual practice that had long been classed as shameful and stigmatised, such as polyamory, porn production, kink, queer sex, sex work and promiscuity.

However, there have been limitations to the sex positivity movement. As one old member of the 1960s counterculture, David Cooper, argued: "MAKING LOVE IS GOOD IN ITSELF AND THE MORE IT HAPPENS IN ANY WAY POSSIBLE OR CONCEIVABLE BETWEEN AS MANY PEOPLE AS POSSIBLE MORE AND MORE OF THE TIME, SO MUCH THE BETTER.'[14] Is this true?

In the words of Ginger who is both asexual and trans nonbinary: 'Most people who use "sex positive" use it to mean "sex is a Good Thing." This can leave people feeling isolated or excluded.'[15] Sometimes, clearly, sex is not a good thing. In the aftermath of the #MeToo revelations, an article in *The Week* magazine went viral online titled, 'The Female Price of Male Pleasure' with the opening sentence: 'The world is disturbingly comfortable with the fact that women sometimes leave a sexual encounter in tears.'[16] The piece explored the fact that around 30 per cent of (cis) women experience pain during vaginal sex and 'large proportions' wouldn't tell their partner about it.[17]

Sex can be difficult and painful. Some, like Ginger, are also asexual and have no sexual attraction at all. Sex positive movements, which should be about prioritising consent and communication, have the tendency to tip over into conformity. In an effort to dismantle and challenge heteronormativity, it can come

14   David Cooper, *The Death of the Family* (Harmondsworth, Penguin, 1971), 47–8.
15   https://theestablishment.co/on-being-game-what-happens-when-sex-positivity-feels-like-pressure.
16   https://theweek.com/articles/749978/female-price-male-pleasure.
17   www.ncbi.nlm.nih.gov/pubmed/25648245.

hand in hand with the pressure to be kinky, to be sexually liberated and to have loads of sex all of the time. As we've seen though, this isn't the reality for many people. Being sex positive is also about having the power and agency to say *no*, to have infrequent sex and sometimes having no sex at all – for whatever reason. In the words of Jack and Saff:

Jack, 26

I'm still a virgin and I'm twenty-six. As a teenager I struggled with severe depression and anxiety, which made it near impossible for me to talk to girls. My self-esteem has been extremely low for years and I live at my parents house and it made dating near impossible. I was bullied about it in school about it but honestly I don't care anymore. I'm happy now, and I know there's much more to me than my sex life.

Saff E. D., 21

Honesty. Choice. It all comes down to that. I would describe myself as sex positive. But I'm not less sex positive because I'm a virgin. Or because I want to wait until marriage. People should be allowed to have sex when and with who they want. Stop calling girls sluts and guys studs. Sex positivity is about not having shame where you do or don't. I've heard that in the sixties, a time that was supposed to be liberated, if you didn't have lots of sex people would look down on you and think you're a prude. That's not sex positive – that is coercive. It's about your ability to choose without being negatively affected by whether you have or haven't.

Chapter 8

Sexual violence: 'Abuse of power comes as no surprise'

The rising public concern about rape in the United States has inspired countless numbers of women to divulge their past encounters with actual or would-be assailants. As a result, an awesome fact has come to light: appallingly few women can claim that they have not been victims, at one time in their lives, of either attempted or accomplished sexual attacks.[1] – Angela Davis, 1981

Davis could have been writing in 2017. The phrase Me Too was first used by activist Tarana Burke ten years previously in a campaign to reach underprivileged girls dealing with sexual abuse, but it reached the headlines after allegations of sexual assault within Hollywood led actor Alyssa Milano to send out the following tweet: 'If you've been sexually harassed or assaulted write "me too" as a reply to this tweet.' Within a matter of hours, tens of thousands of people around the world were using the hashtag, confirming what many of us already knew: just how everyday sexual violence really is.

As we saw in Chapter 3, the threat of sexual violence is used to push an agenda against trans people and as we will see later in this

---

1   Angela Davis, *Women, Race and Class* (New York: Vintage Press, 1983).

chapter, remarkably similar rhetoric is occurring at the moment in far-right groups in the UK against Muslim men. The fact that there is still so much shame and silence around sexual violence and an unwillingness to believe survivors[2] has meant that myths and dangerous narratives prevail. So we'll start by answering some basic questions: What is sexual violence? Where does it take place? And finally, I'll give a couple of pointers on how we can support survivors.

What is sexual violence?

Sexual violence is defined as any sexual act directed to a person using coercion and without consent. As we saw in Chapter 5, non-consent is not just limited to physical force, it can also be emotional – for instance intimidation, blackmail, financial threat and emotional manipulation would all be considered a form of coercion. Sexual violence also takes place if someone is *unable* to consent, so if they are drunk or asleep.

A wide range of sexually violent acts can take place in different circumstances and settings. These include, but are not limited to:

- Rape
- Attempted rape
- Fondling or unwanted touching
- Revenge texting or revenge porn
- Sexual trafficking
- Unwanted sexual advances
- Forced marriage or cohabitation
- Denial of the right to use contraception

---

2 Although people differ in what word they prefer to call themselves, I will use 'survivor', rather than 'victim' throughout this chapter. A 'victim' implies passivity and helplessness. 'Survivor' on the other hand gives strength, agency and power back.

- Forced abortion
- Violent acts against sexual integrity, such as Female Genital Mutilation

Sexual harassment is one type of sexual violence and is illegal. According to the UK 2010 Equalities Act, sexual harassment is unwanted behaviour of a sexual nature which: i) violates your dignity; ii) makes you feel intimidated, degraded or humiliated; iii) creates a hostile or offensive environment. Crucially, you do *not* have to have previously objected to someone or their behaviour for it to be unwanted. Behaviours that would be considered harassment include, but are not limited to:

- Someone making sexually degrading comments or gestures
- Being stared or leered at
- Being subjected to sexual jokes or propositions
- Receiving e-mails, messages or texts with sexual content
- Physical behaviour, including unwelcome sexual advances and touching
- Someone displaying sexually explicit pictures in your space or a shared space, like at work or school
- Offers of rewards in return for sexual favours[3]

The personal cost of sexual violence can be devastating. Some of the potential physical side effects include pregnancy (about five per cent of all pregnancies around the world have resulted from rape), STIs and internal trauma. The emotional and mental side effects of sexual violence range from PTSD, to social isolation, depression, anorexia and suicidal behaviour. In many cultures and communities, sexual violence is so stigmatised that it may lead to

---

3 https://rapecrisis.org.uk/get-help/looking-for-information/what-is-sexual-violence/other-kinds-of-sexual-violence/what-is-sexual-harassment/

social stigmatisation, or in extreme cases when pregnancy might be involved, forced marriage.

Where does sexual violence take place?

90 per cent of sexual violence cases take place between people who already know each other. Whether that's a partner, family member, teacher, colleague or carer. The myth of the rapist in the dark alley is precisely that – a myth. The fact that it's often so intimate and personal partly contributes to why sexual violence around the world has been by and large a neglected and misunderstood area of research – data is scarce and fragmented. The main place that records would be collected is through the police, but the overwhelming majority of people do not report sexual violence to police. In the UK, around five in six – approximately 83 per cent – of cases are not reported.[4] This could be due to a number of reasons – to protect the perpetrator, shame, fear or being blamed, not believed or mistreated or in cases involving migrants, there's often a language barrier or fear of deportation.

Sexual violence takes place around the world. However, there are conditions that increase the chances of it taking place. It can be difficult to accept that the most powerful institutions could harbour sexual violence, on an epidemic scale. Hollywood. The Church. Schools. Families. The police. Charities. Government. The Media. They partly maintain their position of power and authority precisely because we trust them and have faith in them. But it's because they have so much power and a lack of accountability that these abuses are able to take place.

Take the workplace as an example. In many instances today, our employers actually hold more power over us than the gov-

---

4   www.ons.gov.uk/peoplepopulationandcommunity/crimeandjustice/articles/sexualoffencesinenglandandwales/yearendingmarch2017.

ernment.[5] They can dictate how we dress, what we're allowed to say on social media, even what we do with our free time. In some workplaces, it is perfectly legal around the world for staff to be refused toilet breaks; for their belongings to be searched when they start and end their days; for their communications to be monitored; to be given forced medical testing or to be fired for their political beliefs.

The earliest records of women's experiences in work situations include complaints of sexual harassment. The Harvey Weinstein scandal has catapulted work-based sexual harassment into the public consciousness. Working in an industry with precarious working conditions, little support and great power imbalances makes women more vulnerable. Weinstein could make or break you in a moment. He had the power to make someone a great acting success. He also had the power to ensure you wouldn't be employed again.

The Democratic Republic of Congo (DRC) is a country notorious for rape being used as a weapon of war – which is true. However, exactly the same proportion of women on US University campuses experience sexual assault or rape as in the DRC. Between one in three and one in four.

Sexual violence is not, as it's often assumed, exclusively about sexual desire or gratification. All research shows that the main motivation behind sexually violent acts is power and control. As the most recent World Health Organization's global report on sexual violence states 'Sexual violence is rather a violent, aggressive and hostile act aiming to degrade, dominate, humiliate, terrorize and control the victim.' Take revenge texting and revenge porn as commonplace examples of sexual violence. What is it about, if it's not to do with subjecting someone to the most extreme public humiliation?

---

5   Elizabeth Anderson, *Private Government: How Employers Rule Our Lives* (Princeton and Oxford: Princeton University Press, 2017).

While anyone of any age, gender and race can be subjected to sexual violence – and we'll cover more of this in the next section on accessing support – sexual violence tends to work on already existing lines of inequality, as these statistics show:

- Women are five times more likely than men to have experienced some type of sexual assault, including unwanted touching or indecent exposure (Office of National Statistics, 2017)
- 46 per cent of bisexual women have been raped, compared to 17 per cent of heterosexual women and 13 per cent of lesbians (NISVS, 2010)
- 40 per cent of gay men and 47 per cent of bisexual men have experienced sexual violence other than rape, compared to 21 per cent of heterosexual men (NISVS, 2010)
- The 2015 U.S. Transgender Survey found that 47 per cent of transgender people are sexually assaulted at some point in their lifetime, compared with five per cent of cis-men.[6]
- Disabled women are twice as likely to be assaulted or raped as non-disabled women (Women's Aid 2007)

Sexual violence is disproportionately gendered and rooted in ideologies of male sexual entitlement. If we understand sexual violence to be about power, domination and control and patriarchal belief systems strip women of the agency to make an autonomous decision about participating in sex, then sexual violence is a savage but necessary end result of patriarchal hierarchies.[7] The link

---

6 www.transequality.org/sites/default/files/docs/USTS-Full-Report-FINAL.PDF.
7   R. Jewkes and K. Wood, '"Dangerous" love: reflections on violence among Xhosa township youth,' In: R. Morrell, ed. *Changing men in Southern Africa* (Pietermaritzburg: University of Natal Press, 2001); R. E. Ariffin, *Shame, secrecy and silence: study of rape in Penang* (Penang: Women's Crisis Centre, 1997); L. Bennett, L. Manderson and J. Astbury, 'Mapping a global pandemic: review of current literature on rape, sexual assault and sexual harassment of women' (Melbourne: University of Melbourne, 2000).

between patriarchal value systems and sexual violence has been made clear over and over again, with all research showing that societies with higher gender inequality have higher frequency of male rape.[8] As we'll see in the next section on accessing support, not all women experience sexual violence in the same way.

Guardian journalist Frances Ryan explains how power and sexual violence operate in relation to disability: 'I don't describe disabled people – including myself – as "vulnerable". It's generally a patronising, pitying sort of comment. It also homogenises a vast, complex group: anyone from a 56-year-old woman who uses a wheelchair to a teenage boy with Down's syndrome. But the uncomfortable truth is that being disabled makes someone vulnerable to abuse: whether that is because a severe learning disability means a victim cannot understand what is happening to them, or because a spinal injury means a woman who is being assaulted cannot sit up. To an abuser who likes power and control, a disability is perfect.'[9]

Supporting survivors

In a culture that disbelieves survivors, taking active steps to listen is crucial to believing survivors. At the back of the book, there's a list of organisations that can be contacted for further support, although it is by no means an exhaustive list.

Not all survivors are the same. In 1991, academic and feminist Kimberlé Williams Crenshaw famously identified the different ways that black and white women experience accessing support after sexual and domestic violence in the US. Drawing on her previous work from 1989, in which she developed the theory of intersectionality she interrogated the ways that class, race and

---

8   P. Sanday, 'The socio-cultural context of rape: a cross-cultural study,' *Journal of Social Issues* 37, (1981): 5–27.
9   www.theguardian.com/commentisfree/2015/may/18/abuse-disabled-people-sexually-abused-england-cuts-services.

gender created different access needs for women – which needs to be considered to support survivors.

Crenshaw showed that many women of colour in the US (and globally although this was not her focus) are disproportionately burdened by poverty and caring responsibilities and due to institutional racism and sexism, struggle to access the job market. She spoke about women who have precarious immigration status and were subsequently reluctant to leave even the most abusive partners in case they are deported. There are language barriers that can limit the possibility of non-English speaking women to access mainstream domestic violence and sexual violence support. In the words of bell hooks, Crenshaw 'challenged the notion that "gender" was the primary factor determining a woman's fate'.[10]

It's crucial that class and race are considered when support for survivors is given. While sexual violence is disproportionately gendered, it's clear that it's not just women who are affected. It's estimated that one in six men have been abused before the age of sixteen, but the figure may be much higher since a whopping 96 per cent of sexual offences against males go unreported.[11] I spoke to Ross Phillips, a psychologist from the Male Survivors Partnership in Manchester, a survivor-led and survivor-run organisation that supports male survivors of sexual abuse and rape:

Amongst all survivors there's a culture of shame, guilt and secrecy, but in my experience I've seen this most acutely amongst men. The most important barrier to giving people the support they need is the secrecy around abuse – so shame becomes a big problem. While it is getting better, there is still shame around male rape, and it means there's not nearly enough research or

10   bell hooks, *Feminist Theory: From Margin to Center*, third edition (New York: Routledge, 2014).

11   glaconservatives.co.uk/wp-content/uploads/2015/11/Silent-Suffering.pdf.

funding. I have some clients that travel over two hours to visit me on a weekly basis.

The culture of shame and silence among male survivors requires particular care and support. And, as Crenshaw famously argued in 1991, women of colour's access needs are different to white women's. As anyone that works in the field of supporting survivors will tell you – far more research, education and funding is needed to give the scale of tailored support to tackle the complexity and pervasiveness of sexual violence.

Tommy Robinson

Stephen Yaxley-Lennon has a new life purpose. Like a white knight, his mission is to take on sexual violence; to root out perpetrators of heinous crimes and protect helpless victims. But this isn't his first quest. Back in 2009 Yaxley-Lennon set up an organisation called the English Defence League (EDL), to wash away Islamic extremism from the pure shores of this nation. His organisation did not do well. His ambitions were largely rejected and they were so unpopular that thousands took to the streets to make it known that the EDL and their views were not welcome. In 2013, Yaxley-Lennon jumped the ELD ship, in the hope that he'd find a happy home with a more respectable group. Yaxley-Lennon is a shape-shifter. He's been Andrew McMaster, Paul Harris and Wayne King at different points, but today he is Tommy Robinson, the figurehead of the far right in Britain.

Robinson claims that sexual violence is at the heart of the Muslim Community. He blames the 'liberal elite' for hiding the violence at the heart of Islam, blinded by hypocritical 'tolerance' and faith in multiculturalism and presents himself as the crusader of truth and justice. In May 2018, Robinson was jailed for 13 months for filming outside a rape trial involving defendants of mainly Pakistani heritage. Hundreds of thousands of people watched him talk on an online streamed video for more than an hour about Muslims and 'jihad rape gangs', before he was taken away by police and charged with contempt of court. Back in 2017 he was found guilty of a similar offence outside Canterbury Court.

Sexual violence is expression of power and domination and it is committed by people of every race and every religion. But Robinson is not interested in other high profile paedophile cases that have involved white people, such as the allegations of abuse in football, public school teachers, care workers or BBC presenters. This is about race – and his track record makes it abundantly clear. He's been caught on film saying things like: 'Somalis are backward barbarians'; British Muslims are 'enemy combatants who want to kill you, maim you and destroy you'; and refugees are 'raping their way through the country'. Just like accusations of sexual violence are slung against the trans community, they are deeply embedded within racist stereotypes about men of colour.

'A nameless horror'

Throughout the slave trade, from 1619 to 1865, a staggering 12.5 million people were captured from all over Africa, put onto ships, taken to the New World and set to work. Once they arrived in America, they were sent to a market, where they would be greeted by browsing slave owners, given a price, bargained for and then separated across the US to work on farms, on the land and in homes. Human beings became commodities.

It was essential that colonised subjects came to be understood as less than human for this scale of subjugation to take place and a whole host of characteristics were ascribed onto race. The highest values of the time, of moral and sexual purity, of absolute reason and rationality were afforded to white people, as people of colour came to be understood in opposition: irrational, depraved and driven by the passions. Even though many slave owners considered it their right to rape the women they enslaved, that didn't matter – it was black men who came to be known as having an untameable lust for white women, that would so often tip over into sexual violence.

The trope of the vulnerable, hapless white woman and the predatory black man continued throughout the twentieth century. *The Birth of a Nation* (originally called The Clansmen) arrived on screens in 1915 and was the first major blockbuster movie in history. It has also been called 'the most racist film ever made'. The story unravels between two white American families during the Civil War, one Union, the other Confederate. In spite of deep political frictions, both families unify against the threat of a black rapist on the run, who's bent on having white women. The Ku Klux Klan (KKK) are employed and they successfully hunt down the man.

The Birth of a Nation had real life consequences. Prior to the film's release, the KKK had practically dwindled in size and importance, but its release triggered a revival of the organisation, leading to its peak in 1925 where membership grew into the millions and 50,000 men in white hoods marched through the streets of Washington.

It's not just in the US where racist stereotypes about men of colour and sexual violence exist. Nazi propaganda was teeming with images of the Jewish man hunting down Aryan women, and these tropes were essential in creating this idea that Jews were a threat to the German nation and people. Robinson's accusations are in this lineage. By preying on the fragility of white masculinity, on racist ideas about the threat of men of colour and the passivity and sexual availability of women, he has tapped into old stereotypes that run deep in Western culture. As history shows, and as I'm sure Robinson is aware – these fears have the power to mobilise a movement.

#METOO

Sexual violence might be as old as time, but so is resistance. For as long as people have abused power, there has always been push back. From the early 1900s, women formed labour unions that fought for the rights of female workers, including the right not to be sexually harassed. In the US, black women's struggles against workplace harassment led to the creation of the first laws against sexual discrimination and harassment. Today, union organising in the lowest paid and most precarious work in the economy, such as outsourced cleaning, are building momentum and winning struggles to improve conditions. Workers in these jobs, which are so often migrant women, might take place at night, with irregular working hours, with little contact of other workers, are rife with stories of harassment and sexual violence. They are also the people that got left behind in the MeToo movement.

Opening up these conversations, challenging abuse, listening and believing people and supporting survivors is essential. As Ross Phillips told me from Male Survivors Partnership in Manchester:

> The most important thing, I believe, that we have to do to tackle sexual violence is to challenge the shame and silence. It's about telling someone: 'this random guy is sending me dick picks, what do I do?' Or 'I have a bad gut feeling about this person, what shall I do'. Always trust your gut. So many people I see at the support centre say that they had a nasty feeling about that person, well before anything happened. It's about listening to that nagging instinct that something is wrong. Always tell someone, no matter how small it seems – because these can be the early signs of abuse.

There have been huge strides, not least in the explosion of stories that #MeToo unearthed. Alicia Garza, one of the co-creators of

Black Lives Matter, and a survivor of sexual assault, gives us hope. She said that the strength of the movement lies in the 'power of empathy, this power of connection, is really about empowering people to be survivors, to be resilient, and also to make really visible that sexual violence is not about people's individual actions, that this is a systemic problem'. I witnessed the power of the campaign firsthand in a conversation I had with a young woman from East London:

Faz 17

I learned so much from the #MeToo movement. I learned way more online than from lessons in schools. I had no idea what consent was before, but now I feel like I can put up boundaries. A lot of religious speakers would never talk about this kind of thing. There is no way I would get my sex ed from them. I learned almost everything I know from the hashtag #MeToo. One thing that's really stuck out to me – I still think it's so crazy – that you just expect people at the age of 30 or 40 would understand consent – but MeToo showed me that they don't. Even after everything though, I still have a lot of hope for the future and my generation.

Chapter 9

Sexuality: From Stonewall to Yarl's Wood

I left home at age ten in 1961. I hustled on 42nd Street. The early 60s was not a good time for drag queens, effeminate boys or boys that wore makeup like we did. Back then we were beat up by the police, by everybody. We expected nothing better than to be treated like we were animals – and we were.

In 1969, the night of the Stonewall riot was a very hot, muggy night. We were in the Stonewall [bar] and the lights came on. We all stopped dancing. The police came in and we were led out of the bar and they cattled us all up against the police vans. The cops pushed us up against the grates and the fences. People started throwing pennies, nickels, and quarters at the cops. And then the bottles started.

I remember when someone threw a Molotov cocktail, I thought: 'My god, the revolution is here. The revolution is finally here!'

I am proud of myself as being there that night. If I had lost that moment, I would have been kind of hurt because that's when I saw the world change for me and my people.

Of course, we've still got a long way ahead of us.

Looking back years later, Sylvia Rivera, a Latina American gay liberation and transgender rights activist, gave this account of the Stonewall riots. Tensions between the LGBTQ+ community and the police had been building well before 28 June 1969. Night after night, police routinely raided the Stonewall Inn, a gay club in Greenwich Village in New York. Sometimes they would make arrests, at other times they'd simply turn up, intimidate people and demand pay-offs in return for not publicly releasing names. This was 1969 in America: being outed could be catastrophic.

The law was not on the side of the Stonewall partygoers. In 1969 it was illegal to serve alcohol to gay people, and it was also illegal for gay men to dance together. There was also the notorious 'three-article rule', which said that people couldn't wear more than three pieces of clothing that didn't match their assigned gender. Sylvia and many others who spent time at Stonewall were trans and were routinely preyed on by the police.

On 28 June 1969 there were about 200 people in the bar and it looked like it would be the usual raid. Within minutes though, hundreds of people had congregated outside the Inn. The police cleared everyone out by 4am but by the next evening over 1,000 people had gathered. The riots would last for days, leading to mass arrests and the closure of the Stonewall Inn. But with this insurrectionary outburst, something had changed that could not be undone. In the months and years following the riots, there was an explosion of gay activism, new political organisations and pride.

It marked a historical turning point for an emboldened gay liberation movement.

Orientation

In the 50 years since the Stonewall riots, a lot has changed. In the UK, an increasing number of people identify as LGBTQ+, with 50 per cent of young people claiming that they do not identify as

'100 per cent heterosexual'.[1] In the United States, there's a similar upward trend, with 14 per cent of young people between the ages of 18 to 34 identifying as LGBTQ+. Such large numbers of young people who feel safe to declare that they are 'not 100 per cent heterosexual' reflects a far more tolerant society than the one the Stonewall rioters were facing back in 1969. These hard-won changes – in law and in attitudes – should not be taken lightly. They've come about as a result of struggle, sacrifice and solidarity.

There has always been dissidence: people acting in defiance against governments, religious institutions and playground bullies to have the right and freedom to love and desire whoever they want. However, in spite of massive steps towards greater tolerance and respect, we do not live in a world that has rid itself of homophobia and queerphobia. The position that heterosexuality is the *de facto* way that humans express their sexuality has deep and strong roots. It is reiterated and reinforced everywhere, in schools, in media, in families, in government and in religious institutions – there is no escaping the fact that today, in the words of Silvia Rivera, 'we've still got a long way ahead of us'.

Sex labs

So what do we know about human sexuality?

The first major comprehensive laboratory study into sexual behaviour came from the controversial but hugely influential American biologist and sexologist Alfred Kinsey. Born in 1894, Kinsey was working in an extremely sexually conservative and cautious era and the kinds of questions he was concerned about went against the grain of almost every value around sex that American society held so dear. Uninhibited from religious and societal norms, he wanted to truly understand what human

---

1   https://yougov.co.uk/topics/lifestyle/articles-reports/2015/08/16/half-young-not-heterosexual.

sexuality was all about. Kinsey initially applied to conduct his research in a university but was repeatedly rejected. So, he resorted to doing research in secret. Kinsey sought out sex workers, prisoners and the underground gay world. He made friends with them and then, often over a cigarette, would propose that they take part in his 'study'. In the end, his small team interviewed approximately 18,000 Americans about their sex lives. The first research entailed 30 couples – some heterosexual and some homosexual – filmed and observed having sex in his attic. His findings about male sexuality were published in 1948 and there was a later study on women in 1953. Both works became national bestsellers, catapulting Kinsey to fame and providing the moral framework – some have argued – for the sexual liberation movements of the sixties.

Today his findings are common knowledge but at the time the results were groundbreaking. His most famous take away was that human sexuality operates on a scale, and not as a binary. He estimated that only 10 per cent of people were completely heterosexual or homosexual, but that the overwhelming majority of us are somewhere in the middle. He also found that sexuality changes throughout the human lifetime. Of the people he interviewed, between 30 to 45 per cent of people had had an extra-marital affair; 37 per cent of men have had a homosexual experience and 17 per cent of farm boys have had intercourse with animals. Kinsey declared that: 'the only unnatural sex act is that which you cannot perform.'

Kinsey used his results to ridicule the existing sex laws in the US. When he was working, sodomy was illegal in many states, as was oral sex. Kinsey pointed out that according to his findings 90 per cent of the male population and 80 per cent of the female population should therefore be in prison. Kinsey was labelled a pervert. He was called a Communist, bent on destroying traditional American family values. His personal life was splashed across the media, stories circulating about his open marriage and his relationships with male students. It was even revealed that he liked to do his gardening wearing nothing but a tight thong.

Kinsey wasn't alone in being attacked for trying to open the door and debunk conservative myths about sexuality. Before the rise of the Nazi party, Berlin was home to the Institute for Sexual Science, a research institute where people could receive free sex advice, treatment for STIs and other sexual problems, and which boasted a library containing the largest collection of literature on sex in the world and a museum stuffed with fetish props. The laboratory employed scientists experimenting to create aphrodisiacs, anti-impotence treatment and even supervised the very first sex reassignment surgery in the world. And yet, the institute was run by Jewish people and communists. So when Hitler rose to power, it was swiftly shut down. The museum was vandalised, files were burned, exhibition cases were smashed and the scientists were forced to flee Germany.

Kinsey told us what many people have always known. That while heterosexuality is prioritised before other sexual expressions, everything else – from history to science, to biology, to zoology to psychology – tells us that human sexuality is fluid, subject to change and anything but simple.

More recent research has developed his work. We know that sexual orientation is not necessarily aligned to your gender; in other words, if you're a cis-woman, it does not necessarily follow that you will only be attracted to cis-men. Writers of queer theory, such as Eve Kosofsky Sedgwick, have argued that any attempt to put sexual desire onto gender or sex is wrong. Calling someone gay implies that they are a cis-man attracted to cis-men. Or a lesbian is a cis-woman attracted to cis-women. Queer theory allows a far more inclusive and fluid notion of gender and sexuality, encompassing the positions of trans, intersex and gender-queer identifying people.

While most people will remember their first crush, that tingling moment of first sexual awakening, around one in a hundred people will have a different memory: a dawning moment of realisation that they still have no attraction to anyone; that they are asexual.

Swinging sixties

Some of Kinsey's methods have been called into question (not least his and his wife's own involvement in some of the more explicit research) but his thesis about the fluidity of human sexuality has been proved right many times. The implications are clear and inclusive. With a politics of consent, they validate the experiences of everyone's own unique and particular sexuality – from asexuality to pansexuality to being queer.

Why must we fight for the commemoration of LGBTQ+ history? Perhaps the answer seems obvious. But just as the Nazi party was desperate to burn and destroy Berlin's institute of Sexology, there are also those that want to forget the history of LGBTQ+ resistance, to purge it and further the idea that heterosexuality is the *de facto* mode of being. Yet by reclaiming and remembering the resistance stories of the past, we can challenge intolerance today.

Male homosexuality has been targeted for centuries in the UK. The Buggery Act of 1533, passed by Parliament during the reign of Henry VIII, marked the first time in the UK that male homosexuality was legally targeted for persecution. It criminalised male sodomy not only in Britain, but also, one day, throughout the whole British Empire, which would come to cover a third of the planet. Convictions were punishable by death. But persecution doesn't trump sexuality. Peter Ackroyd's history of queer London shows that a male brothel even existed on the present site of Buckingham Palace.[2]

---

2   Ackroyd, Peter, *Queer City: Gay London from Romans to the Present Day* (London: Chatto & Windus, 2018).

In London the official punishment for sodomy was death by fire. Yet prosecutions were rare. The law said that it had to be witnessed, and penetration proved. It wasn't until the Victorian era that private sex acts were included and banned, and there was a serious attempt to crack down on so-called 'deviant' sexualities. Public parks were locked at night. Executions for sodomy peaked, and 80 men were hanged over 30 years. Other offenders had mud dumped on them, emblematic of the links between homosexuality and excrement. The story goes, that lesbian sex was also due to be criminalised in this legislation, until Queen Victoria herself intervened and prevented it from being included. She declared that there was no such thing – because it was physically impossible for two women to have sex. As compelling as this myth is, it's likely that it's apocryphal. It was the case that in England around this time a common joke was that lesbianism only existed in France, 'a time when lurid, fictionalised lesbianism was often figured as an especially repulsive/seductive French vice'.[3]

The reality is that the history of the UK and other Western nations is not one championing LGBTQ+ rights. Alan Turing was the English man who is credited for cracking the German 'Enigma' code – the highly advanced German encoding device that allowed messages to be sent across the world without interception. His work cut World War Two short by two years, thus saving millions of lives. Turing's work helped set the foundations for developing an invention that has transformed the world: the modern computer. Despite these achievements, in 1952 Turing was arrested after the police discovered that he was having a relationship with another man. After pleading guilty, he agreed to undergo chemical castration and take hormones intended to 'cure' his homosexuality, rather than serve time inside. The pills he was given caused him to grow breasts and made him impotent. By 1954, Alan Turing was found dead from cyanide poisoning, next to

---

3   www.vam.ac.uk/content/articles/s/sex-and-sexuality-19th-century.

a half-eaten apple on his bedside table (it is rumoured that Apple's logo on our iPhones and Macbooks is a reference to Turing).

Not gay as in happy

With changes in law came attitudinal changes. In 2012, approximately 28 per cent of British populations thought that homosexuality is always or mostly wrong. There's been huge progress, since in 1983, 72 per cent of British populations believed it was always or mostly wrong.[4]

Hapsa, 17

There was one guy in the year above who was gay and he was very open about it. We all bullied him and he left the school because of it. I get why he did it. At our school we're 90 per cent or more Muslim Bangladeshi and our community and families were talking about it. It's really hard to be accepted.

John, 19

Attending an all-boys Catholic school in Ireland, my experience of sex education was almost non-existent. When I was around 13, we started a very small topic of sex education in religion and, from what they taught, I grasped the overall message that sex was for a man and woman that were in a loving marriage with the purpose to be child-bearing. I started questioning my sexuality when I began secondary school. Accepting my sexuality was extremely hard for me. Throughout school I spent a lot of time trying to convince myself that I wasn't gay – I didn't tell my family until a couple months ago. Everyone was very supportive in general however I found that I didn't really need support.

4 www.bsa.natcen.ac.uk/latest-report/british-social-attitudes-30/personal-relationships/homosexuality.aspx.

Hapsa and John come from two different religious backgrounds – Muslim and Catholic – and there are different implications and experiences that result from that. But the same is also true of people from non-religious backgrounds. Contemporary French writer Edouard Louis compares being called a 'faggot' in rural France as a kid to the stigmata, the 'marks they'd carve with a red-hot iron or knife' into the bodies of deviant individuals, people who posed a threat to their communities. In the ultra-conservative Russian republic Chechnya, hundreds of gay men have gone missing in recent years. That includes Zelimkhan Bakayev, a well-known singer who left his home in 2017 in Moscow on his way to his sister's wedding in Grozny, Chechnya's capital, and has not been seen since. The police denied this and refused to investigate his whereabouts. It's widely understood that he was killed in Chechnya's crackdown on gay people. The 2018 elections saw Brazilian leader, Jair Bolsonaro, step into office. In 2010 he said: 'I would be incapable of loving a homosexual child. I'm not going to act like a hypocrite here: I'd rather have my son die in an accident than show up with some moustachioed guy. For me, he would have died'.

Rampant homophobia anywhere in the world is inexcusable. Nonetheless today sexual tolerance is understood as the cornerstone of Western democracies – and is used as a way to justify military action against other states. In 2011, David Cameron threatened withholding aid from countries where homosexuality was illegal. The treatment of LGBTQ+ people in Russia has rightly outraged Western heads of states. But it has also been used to justify hostile military tactics/further attacks against Russia. The inexcusable persecution of LGBTQ+ people in countries in the Global South, in particular, is also often used to justify forms of neo-colonialism, and a sense of Western moral superiority that can have racist undertones.

Not only does intolerance still run deep throughout British society, with hate crime against queer people happening daily, but when we look back at the recent actions of the British government it's clear that their hands are far from clean. As recently as 1987, Margaret Thatcher told the Conservative Party conference that 'Children who need to be taught to respect traditional moral values are being taught that they have an inalienable right to be gay'. In the context of a media storm about AIDS, or the 'gay-bug' as it was also so-called, Section 28 was introduced which made it illegal for local councils to 'promote homosexuality'. That included schools in sex education. Astonishingly, the act was only repealed in 2003.

There are still challenges for most LGBTQ+ people, but for those that have other kinds of privilege – whether that's race, wealth or class – it's undeniably a different kind of struggle. Today the UK government detains more than 27,000 people in immigration detention centres, many of whom are fleeing persecution for being gay or gender non-conforming. The Home Office has been known to use methods to prove the sexuality of some asylum seekers, including extremely explicit questioning, and insisting that evidence is provided.[5] Additionally, according to Home Office figures released in 2017, of 3,535 asylum claims[6] related to sexuality over a two-year period, a staggering two-thirds were rejected. In many instances people are deported back to countries that are notorious for their punitive laws on sexuality. Those in power may support some queer people, but there are still forms of deep homophobia at the heart of the government's immigration policies.

Stonewall's legacy is key. Their fight was not just about LGBTQ+ rights, it was also a challenge to brutal policing, to poverty and

5   https://uklgig.org.uk/?page_id=1225.
6   www.telegraph.co.uk/news/2018/01/25/tests-prove-gay-asylum-seekers-telling-truth-sexuality-break.

to laws that profited some at the expense of others. It was about transformational societal change and connecting their struggle to others. The early LGBTQ+ movement was bound by a politics of solidarity, and it had strong links to the hyper-masculine trade union movements of the time, to the Black Panther Party in the US and to Women's Liberation movements. As the old saying goes, injustice anywhere is a threat to justice everywhere.

Chapter 10

Pornography: Sex education today

If we invent a machine, the first thing we are going to do – after making a profit – is use it to watch porn. – Damon Brown, *Playboy* magazine writer

In porn-speak, if you find yourself under Mark Spiegler's wing then you've made it. 'The Spiegler Girls' triumph at every major porn awards ceremony, they make higher wages than anyone else and there's a steady flow of work. In the words of Spiegler 'companies book them because these girls are professional. They show up on time with their [health] tests and ID. I tell the girls, 'You have three jobs.' The first, he says, is to have sex on camera. The second and third: 'Don't make me look bad, and don't give me something to worry about.'[1] The Spiegler Girls listen to him: since he founded the talent agency in 2003, only one performer has ever been late to a shoot.[2]

Mark Spiegler's story is not common. Since the proliferation of free porn, most performers can only dream about this kind of job security. Whereas at the turn of the century, the average female porn performer was making around $100,000 a year, today that

---

1 www.ibtimes.com/bed-porn-super-agent-mark-spiegler-its-business-sex-1792720.
2 Ibid.

figure is closer to $50,000.[3] The rate is even lower for performers of colour.[4] Rising job precariousness and stagnating wages is not a problem unique to the porn industry. The shift towards a 'gig economy' – where people work from gig to gig, rather than having full stable employment – is visible across sectors. These changes are especially felt in jobs held by the working classes, women, people of colour and the young. The thing that makes porn different from a cafe or bar job though is simple: it's taboo and it's underground.

Watching porn is laced with shame. It would certainly not be the go-to topic to bring up with your family or even friends, but as all statistics shows it is a fundamental part of the private lives of billions of people around the world. People watch porn for all manner of reasons. They watch it alone, with partners, in cinemas, on mobiles and at home. But for around 60 per cent of young people in the UK, porn is also watched to learn about sex.[5] When over half of eleven to thirteen-year-olds have seen porn before starting secondary education and 60 per cent have watched it by the age of 14, it's clear that for plenty of even younger people, pornography is their *first*, and sometimes only, schooling on sex.

Learning from porn is not the same as watching it for pleasure. In this chapter, we'll look at what porn teaches, and we'll consider how it might be related to changes to the porn industry.[6] I'll be focussing primarily on the porn that most people watch – free, mainstream, commercial and for heterosexual consumption.

---

3   www.businessinsider.com/heres-what-female-porn-stars-get-paid-for-different-types-of-scenes-2012-11?r=US&IR=T.

4   Dr. Mireille Miller-Young, *A Taste for Brown Sugar: Black Women in Pornography* (Durham: Duke University Press, 2014).

5   www.nus.org.uk/en/news/students-turn-to-porn-to-fill-the-gaps-in-their-sex-education.

6   For the majority of this, we'll be talking about mainstream, mass consumed and free heterosexual pornography, since that categorises by far the most porn online. At the end of the chapter, however, I'll go over some of the alternatives.

However, at the end of the chapter we'll go over the alternative types.

Searchable terms

The first known piece of pornography is angelic by today's standards. Found in 1908 on the banks of the Danube river in Austria, the 'Venus of Willendorf' is a pocket-sized stone carving of a faceless and curvaceous woman, approximately 25,000 years old. With heavy breasts, over-exaggerated genitals and a swollen backside, it's understood that The Venus is a prime example of a fertility fetish. It's highly unlikely that her body shape would make it to the top of most RedTube searches today, but The Venus was also created into a completely different world. Her creators were nomadic hunter-gatherers living in the midst of Europe's last ice age. They roamed the land, searching for food and shelter, all the while enduring a bleak and hostile world. Where basic survival was a daily grind, scattered communities depended on highly fertile women.

Porn might be as old as time, but it wasn't until the mid-twentieth century, when obscenity laws relaxed and the popularity of magazines like *Playboy* and *Hustler* boomed, that the industry commercialised and exploded in size. When these magazines were first around in the sixties and seventies, porn was pricey and hard to find – today it is instantly and freely accessible. Tech got its teeth into porn and changed it beyond recognition. With smartphones glued to our side and never far from a laptop or computer, we now have unprecedented and limitless access to smut. It's estimated that 14 per cent of all online searches are pornographic, leading some to say that 'the Internet was made for porn'. Pornhub alone attracts more than 80 million visitors a day.

The move towards free porn was inevitable. From YouTube to iPlayer, readily available free visual content – legal and illegal

– exploded in the 'naughties'. However, the way that free porn would turn out was not predictable and many put the responsibility on the shoulders of one man – Fabian Thylmann, also known as 'the man who made porn free'. In 2010, Thylmann started the company Manwin, which swiftly bought up Pornhub, YouPorn, RedTube, Brazzers, twistys.com and other free porn websites. Within two years of establishing Manwin, by Thylmann's estimations, 80 per cent of everyone who watched porn was watching it through one of his sites. In 2013, 65 to 75 million people were using his websites every single day.

Free porn blew all competition out the water. Where the industry was once dominated by large porn production companies, new individual users could now upload their own content far faster and in far greater volume than anything the old producers could compete with. The old-style larger and more expensive shoots became almost untenable in comparison to the DIY, cheap or 'gonzo' stuff. Today, it's believed that 95 per cent of all current productions are gonzo shoots.

The surge in free porn has impacted workers' rights, but it has also impacted the kinds of porn that we consume. In the podcast series the 'Butterfly Effect', psychologist and author Jon Ronson investigated these effects. He interviewed porn performers, producers, consumers and the new tech workers who had written the code to make the proliferation of so much free porn not only possible but also unprecedentedly successful. The majority of these employees worked in Montreal, Canada – a long way from California's San Fernando Valley, where most of the world's porn is made – and they had never, Ronson shows, stepped foot on a porn set in their life. What they were good at was tech, number crunching, hard data and figuring out the right algorithms to get people coming back for more and more. They would track the spikes in usages of websites, noting whether they were watched on phones or computers, at what time, for how long and – importantly here – what people wanted to watch.

Ronson shows that the most important impact of free porn hasn't been increased violence – as many like to argue – but keywords. Everything has to be searchable by a particular category, and these keywords have been chosen as a result of the painstaking testing and data analysis – the kind of scrutiny and research that the old companies (who didn't have an army of Ivy League computer science graduates working for them) were not undertaking. Having an industry that's now dictated by keywords and categories means that performers are living between the terms. Women in their mid-twenties are falling between the cracks – between those don't fit being either 'teen' or 'milf' or mother-age. In the words of one producer Ronson interviews, 'they're just attractive and "just attractive" isn't a searchable term.'

It's a disgrace!

Jasmin, 25

I'm really open with my family about sex. My Mum's Colombian and she absolutely hates when I talk about sex, she's always telling me to shut up . . . but anyway, I really think it's so important. I'm always talking to my brother about sex and girls. The other day I just said to him, if there's one thing you need to know about porn is that it's not real. I didn't want to tell him not to watch it, I wouldn't take that away from him. Everyone needs a release – we all get cranky! But he just has to know that it's not real and that women won't be like they are in porn. He needs to learn this early.

As Jasmin has explained to her younger brother, porn is not reality; it's a performance. It's no secret that there are impossible

121

and unreachable standards in heterosexual mainstream porn and questionable representation of people. Most of the time, cis-male pleasure takes centre stage – queer, lesbian sex is unrealistic and for the enjoyment of the male onlooker. Then there are the unreachable standards of beauty and sexual performance, for all genders. Consent is rarely given. Trans people are assumed to be de-facto 'kinky'; it's highly unlikely that you will see someone with visible disabilities; and your average porn site is littered with racial stereotypes. Black men are depicted as sexual predators with larger than average penises. It won't take long on a porn homepage before you will see degrading stereotypes about women of colour, like 'Dominating Ebony', 'Latina Housemaid' and 'Submissive Asian Babes'.

As we'll see again in the following chapter on dating, when these sexualised stereotypes are taken uncritically and unchallenged, they have real life effect. It's degrading and dehumanising if you're on the receiving end of misogyny, yellow or jungle fever or any other kind of discrimination, whether or not said to you swaddled with 'it's just my preference, I can't help that I like [insert racial stereotype]'. The fetishisation of Asian woman, in particular, is so pervasive in porn that when you type in Google Images 'Asian', some of the first photographs to come up will be pornographic. If you have the urge to do the same with 'European', you'll be confronted with a profoundly unsexy stream of pictures of the European Union flag.

But we know this – and it's partly why there's so much shame and guilt attached to porn. The question is how to deal with it. Most people have strong opinions about sexual behaviour, and porn seems to bring out the strongest of those strong opinions. When it comes to the question of young people and pornography in the press, there is nothing short of moral panic.

- 'SICKENING STATS Experts blame online porn as shocking figures reveal one Scottish child is charged with rape or attempted rape EVERY WEEK,' *Sun*, 2017
- 'The scary effects of pornography: how the 21st century's acute addiction is rewiring our brains,' *Telegraph*, 2017
- 'Children aged 8 addicted to online pornography,' *Daily Mail*, 2012
- 'Sexual Violence is the new normal in India – and pornography is to blame, *Guardian*, 2018

Since the rise of online porn, discussions within the media have taken on a life of their own. They are highly emotive, scaremongering and most of the time unhinged from a credible evidence base. Much like it's near impossible to say what the effect of playing video games are on the mind, there's very little conclusive evidence on the effects of porn. Specifically here, there is no conclusive evidence to say that watching porn makes the viewer more violent.

The Conservative Party in the UK is absolutely clear on their position. To them, porn is a force for social ill – it is corrupting for the youth, it is damaging for women and it must be controlled. In 2013, British Prime Minister David Cameron's government made public that it was their intention to crack down on the industry and thus 'protect women from harm'.[7]

---

7 This was all without even a hint of self-awareness. High ranking Tories are notorious for their insatiable appetite for pornography. Within years of Cameron's statement, Damian Green, the ex-Secretary for State was forced to resign after police found thousands upon thousands of pornographic images on his work computer. These two particular policies were being discussed in the midst of some of the most savage public sector cuts that the UK has ever seen. The effect of this economic programme has been devastating for women. By 2020, men will have borne just 14 per cent of the total burden of welfare cuts, compared with 86 per cent for women. This includes over two thirds of domestic violence shelters which have faced closure under Tory cuts.

A year later in December 2014, the Conservative government successfully passed a flurry of laws to crack down on porn. They had decided to ban certain sex acts from UK-made porn that they believed to be degrading. These included: 'Face Sitting', female ejaculation, spanking, fisting and water-sports – to name a few. Even though these restrictions were put in place, it didn't stop UK viewers from accessing anything made beyond the seas of this island. The policy was met with fierce resistance. Some people argued that it was censorship. Others showed that all of these acts were about female pleasure and that the law was sexist. Campaigners staged a mass protest outside parliament, as they sung the Monty Python song 'Sit On My Face'. Protesters chanted: 'What do we want? Face-sitting! When do we want it? Now!'

The future

Can porn be used for positive educational purposes? Education journalist at the *Guardian* newspaper, Laura McInerney, taught PSHE in secondary schools in East London for six years and believes so. When I spoke to Laura on the phone, she told me that porn had been an important part of her sex ed classes. 'Porn gets pupils asking better questions. Often in my classrooms pupils would challenge something based on the statement 'but that's not how it works in porn'. Or they would begin, 'I saw this thing in a porn clip where . . .' and then ask to understand it more.' Unlike many teachers, Laura moved beyond the awkwardness and they were able to have open and healthy conversations about the gap between porn and real life.

Erika Lust, a well-known Swedish feminist porn filmmaker, is in consultation with sex educators to create a porn-education website for parents. She also argues that at an appropriate age, young people should be introduced to what she calls 'healthy porn', porn that prioritises consent, is queer friendly, celebrates all kinds of sexuality and treats its workers well.

Porn is unstoppable. The industry is already experimenting with Virtual Reality (VR), and there are already developments into so-called 'sex robots' and the 'campaign against sex robots' has also already started. It's estimated that the VR porn industry will be worth one billion dollars by 2025. Porn adapts with the times.

Chapter 11

Sex work: The oldest job in the world

On 4 December 2013 over 200 members of the London Metropolitan riot police stormed and raided the brothels of Soho, London. These were some of the accounts of the workers:

> Forty officers came into our building, approximately 20 went upstairs and 20 came into our flat. They were dressed in full riot gear, with dogs – everything but guns. They broke down our door even though they knew women were inside and even though we had already opened the door to let some police in.

> Both me and the maid were handcuffed and held on the floor and she is in her 70s. What threat are we? They say I am a victim but treat me like a dangerous criminal.

> The police went to my home and searched it. My daughter was there and they told my daughter that I work in Soho and what I do. This was vindictive.

> I am Romanian and I was told by a policeman that I don't have the right to be here. Yes I do. I am a self-employed sex worker and I have the right to live and work here.[1]

---

1 All accounts taken from English Collective of Prostitutes website: http://prostitutescollective.net/2014/01/the-soho-raids-what-really-happened/ (last accessed 11/2018).

Ever since the first brothel opened in Soho in 1778, the area has been known as a noisy, lawless village in the heart of one of the oldest and wealthiest cities in the world. Back in the 1970s when red lights shone from entrances, nearly every other building was either a strip club, massage parlour or sex shop. Unsuspecting passers by found themselves in 'that' part of town, quickly turning back on themselves as they walked past window-displays proudly filled with fetish wear and porn magazines. There was a dark side to Soho. Addiction and drug abuse ran rife, and poor health care and homelessness ran abundant, but accounts from people that lived there say there was also a fierce sense of community and support. Drag kings and queens would party all night long, defiantly protecting each other if there was ever any trouble.

Walk through Soho today and you will see a changed place. Rising rents have pushed out most of the old residents, impossibly expensive wine bars are commonplace and police presence has ensured that the sex trade is out of sight. It's no surprise that Soho has been described as on 'the front line of gentrification'.[2]

What is sex work?

People have sex for all manner of reasons, but for 40–42 million people around the world today, sex is a way to make a living.[3] Sex work can mean a number of things: porn, companionship, domination, stripping and escorting. It can be lucrative and it can be badly paid. It can be safe and it can be dangerous.

Today is a different story. Trafficking and human slavery are very real contemporary phenomena but they are often mistakenly conflated with sex work. While there is no evidence that in the

---

2   www.thetimes.co.uk/article/soho-property-market-london-gentrification-vttd3d66v.
3   www.lefigaro.fr/actualite-france/2012/01/13/01016-20120113ARTFIG00766-40-a-42-millions-de-personnes-se-prostituent-dans-le-monde.php.

UK all women prostitutes are victims of trafficking, this myth is propagated everywhere. Fiona Mactaggart, a former Home Office minister, told BBC Radio 4's *Today in Parliament* in January 2008 that 'something like 80 per cent of women in prostitution are controlled by their drug dealer, their pimp, or their trafficker'.[4] This statistic was repeated everywhere – by former Solicitor General, Vera Baird MP, participants on BBC Radio and in the news. The fact that it was inaccurate didn't seem to matter.

A far more comprehensive and recent study of migrant sex workers found less than 6 per cent had been trafficked. The same study found that in fact the majority of sex workers were not coerced into selling sex but rather chose to work in the sex industry rather than in the 'unrewarding and sometimes exploitative conditions they meet in non-sexual jobs'.[5] To be clear: sex trafficking is a serious problem that deserves attention, campaigning and more than one short chapter written on the subject. Nonetheless, although sex work brings up a whole set of dangers, they are not the same as those that people who are trafficked are affected by. Treating them as the same thing helps no one.

There are important similarities between sex work and other kinds of employment. Consent is paramount to sex work, although in practice it may not always be there. In the words of sex workers and authors of *Revolting Prostitutes*, Molly Smith and Juno Mac, 'Just as forcing a massage therapist to give you oral sex would constitute sexual assault, because she is not giving you the "right" to her body when she sells massage services, forcing a sex worker to (for instance) have sex without a condom constitutes rape precisely because the sex worker has not sold the right for a client to use her body "as he likes in the time he has purchased it".'[6]

---

4   www.theguardian.com/uk/2009/oct/20/trafficking-numbers-women-exaggerated.

5   N. Mai, *Migrant Workers in the UK Sex Industry: ESRC Full Research Report* (2011).

6   Molly Smith and Juno Mac, *Revolting Prostitutes: The Fight for Sex Workers' Rights* (London: Verso, 2018), 111.

SEX WORK: THE OLDEST JOB IN THE WORLD

Throughout history, sex work has been a matter of survival for marginalised groups and today is no different. As Smith and Mac put it, 'People who sell or trade sex are among the world's least powerful people, the people often forced to do the worst jobs.'[7] People of all genders make a living selling sex, but it's important not to lose sight that it is a disproportionately feminised industry.[8] 88 per cent of approximately 72,800 sex workers in the UK are women – both cis and trans[9] – and more than 70 per cent of UK sex workers have previously worked in healthcare, education or the voluntary sector – professions that are similarly dominated by women.[10]

Sex work can be a way to make an income when the wider job market excludes groups of people. In the words of poet and sex worker Pluma Sumaq for many people of colour, 'Prostitution is not what you do when you hit rock bottom. Prostitution is what you do to stay afloat, to swim rather than sink, to defy rather than disappear.'[11] It's estimated that one-quarter of homeless youth in London are LGBTQ+, and of that group around 70 per cent were kicked out by their families.[12] LGBTQ+ are over-represented within the sex industry. Race and disability are also key factors in why people might go into sex work.

People sell sex to make money and people make money to survive. In an effort to highlight that for people in the industry it's

7   Ibid., 129.
8   Ibid., 19.
9   B. Brooks-Gordon, N. Mai, G. Perry and T. Sanders, *Calculating the Number of Sex Workers and Contribution to Non-Observed Economy in the UK* (Office for National Statistics, 2015).
10   P. Sumaq, 'A Disgrace Reserved for Prostitutes: Complicity & the Beloved Community', *LIES: A journal of materialist feminism* (2015), 2, 11–24, 13–14, available at liesjournal.net.
11   P. Sumaq, 'A Disgrace Reserved for Prostitutes: Complicity & the Beloved Community', *LIES: A journal of materialist feminism* 2, (2015): 11–24, 13–14.
12   T. Gorton, 'A quarter of the UK's homeless youth are LGBT', *Dazed*, (27 February 2015).

a job and a way to make money, rather than an identity, there has been an active campaign to try and replace the word 'prostitute' with the term 'sex worker'. Imagine how degrading it would be to be called 'Bartender' every waking moment, even if you're not at work. Or 'Check Out Girl'. Or 'Sales Assistant'. The word prostitute reduces someone to their profession. 'Sex worker' emphasises that it's a job, something you do for a living rather than something that you are.[13]

Sex work may not actually be 'the oldest profession in the world' (as I've called it in the title of this chapter) – midwifery, for instance, is likely far older – but it has been around for a very long time. In Babylonia, Sumaria, and among the Phoenicians, prostitutes were women who had sex as a religious ritual. In the Jewish scriptures Rahab, a prostitute from Jericho, notoriously betrayed her people and assisted the Israelites to capture the city. She tied scarlet rope around her house to identify where she lived – some suggest that this is where the term 'Red Light' comes from. In England, during Tudor times, brothels were immensely popular and syphilis was so widespread, that the term 'goose bumps' emerged as slang for having a VD. In an effort to 'clean' up the country, Henry VIII ordered his government to clamp down on prostitution. He had little success. Not only did his son, Edward VI, open up all establishments again as soon as he took the throne, but some of the brothels outside London were surrounded by treacherous moats and impossibly high walls, preventing the King's forces from entering.

'Protecting women'

With neither drawbridges nor moats, London's Soho sex workers of 2013 were not so lucky. There's no doubt that sex work is dangerous. Some research has shown that it's even the most risky

---

13   Juno Mac and Molly Smith, *Revolting Prostitutes* (London: Verso 2018).

profession in the world, with one global review reporting that 45–75 per cent of sex workers experienced workplace violence over a lifetime.[14] There can be a huge risk of coercion, of sexual violence, of sexual and other physical health issues, of abuse and of exploitation. The key debate today is what can be done to make it safer.

In the UK – as well as most countries around the world – sex work is illegal. However, there are loopholes. So while selling and buying sex might be legal, plenty of things around it are not. Kerb crawling and advertising in phone boxes is illegal and so are brothels (any premises which is being used by more than one worker). But to what extent does the criminalisation of sex work actually protect anyone?

After the Soho raid the police also said that they had been looking for 'victims' to 'take them to safety'. But this is not how the workers saw it. I spoke to Nicki Adams from the English Collective of Prostitutes, a group of sex workers campaigning for decriminalisation and safety:

> Soho was one of the safest places that women could work. Sex workers were very integrated into the community and had the support of the rest of the community. So it was a unique place in many ways but also the flats were open door flats, so if you had any trouble you didn't have to worry. Women described that if they got into trouble they would just hang out the window and shout and people would come and help.

During the 2013 raid, the police were accompanied by a troop of UK Border Agency (UKBA) officers and an entourage of journalists, who snapped away feverishly, taking photos. When the papers were printed the next day, they showed women being dragged into

---

14   K. N. Deering, A. Amin, J. Shoveller, A. Nesbitt, C. Garcia-Moreno, P. Duff, E. Argento and K. Shannon, *A Systemic Review of the Correlates of Violence Against Sex Workers* (2014).

the cold London night, covering their faces as they tried to protect their identities. In the words of one:

> I was taken out of the flat in my underwear. It was only because a neighbour from upstairs gave me a cardigan that I had anything on at all. Was this to humiliate me and make a show for the cameras? And I was freezing. Other women weren't given a chance to collect their coats so they were outside in the cold.[15]

In China, police have forced arrested sex workers to parade, handcuffed, in the streets while they were being photographed.[16] While the economy in Greece in 2012 was collapsing, the police staged raids on brothels, under the guise of attempting to rescue 'migrant victims of sex trafficking'. They detained sex workers, made them have HIV tests and then released the results of the tests and photographs of the workers to the media. Melissa Gira Grant, author of *Playing the Whore* asks: 'What more clear signal do we need that the police are more interested in exposing these women than "saving" them? How is their safety compromised now by these images and their spread online, as well?'

A study conducted by the Sex Workers Project in New York found that 30 per cent of sex workers had been threatened with violence by police officers, while 27 per cent actually experienced violence at the hands of police.[17] Around the world, sex workers say the same. Kay Thi Win, a sex worker in Burma, has said: 'We live in daily fear of being "rescued". The violence happens when feminist rescue organisations work with the police, who break

---

15 All accounts taken from English Collective of Prostitutes website: http://prostitutescollective.net/2014/01/the-soho-raids-what-really-happened (last accessed 11/2018).

16 Melissa Gira Grant, *Playing the Whore: the Work of Sex Work* (London: Verso 2014).

17 J. Thukral and M. Ditmore, 'Sex Workers Project at the Urban Justice Center,' *Revolving Door: An Analysis of Street-based Prostitution in New York City* (2003).

into our workplaces and beat us, rape us and kidnap our children in order to save us.'[18]

Police operations are particularly pernicious when they target migrant sex workers. Migrant sex workers are among the most vulnerable to exploitative working conditions and violence (particularly those with an irregular migration status). With the looming threat of detention and deportation, the police force will never be a benevolent or approachable institution. Since the law pushes the trade underground, it actually makes the industry *less* safe, a fact that has not gone unnoticed. Amnesty International, Human Rights Watch and many other groups are all fiercely critical of the UK's treatment of sex workers, and migrant sex workers in particular.

The law makes sex work less safe, but so do societal attitudes. In spite of the long history of prostitution, there is still an enormous stigma attached to sex work. This unmistakably stems from the double standards placed on the shoulders of female sexuality, as we spoke about in Chapter 7 on virginity and purity. In the words of Love Island's Megan Barton-Hanson, who worked as a stripper for years: 'Guys will go out and sleep with loads of girls and get applauded but if a girl dances in her underwear she's called a "slut" and made out to be the biggest slag ever.' Part of the effort to 'save women' is connected to a historical effort to control and shame women. It is men, incidentally, who are more likely to use sex workers, for sex and for emotional support, yet also sling insults like 'whore', 'slag' or 'prostitute' at women who are deemed to be impure.

Decrim now!

Sex work is not safe, but the way sex workers are treated by the state puts them in a more dangerous position. Rather than

---

18   www.theguardian.com/commentisfree/2013/dec/11/soho-police-raids-sex-workers-fear-trafficking.

deciding for sex workers what's best *for* them and how to save *them*, it's time to listen to the demands they have put forward. Around the world, sex workers and many leading international human rights organisations, including the UN, Amnesty, the World Health Organisation and the World Bank support the full decriminalisation of sex work, removing all laws and policies that criminalise sex work – including selling, buying, and organising. They argue that sex workers should be given the status of a worker, and afforded the same rights that other workers are given, like sick pay, holiday pay, maternity leave and so on.

That said, after long consultations with sex workers, New Zealand became the first country in the world to decriminalise sex work. All the evidence shows that this has brought about many positive benefits for workers, including allowing them to speak more openly about specifically what problems they face and getting more support from health workers, police and others. Some reports have shown that New Zealand's legislation has also been successful in reducing the harms associated with the industry, and that with criminalisation comes greater harm and violence.[19,20]

Simple as the demand for decriminalisation may seem, it is extremely controversial. Many people interpret sex workers' attempts to collectively organise as a way – conscious or not – to encourage others to become sex workers. This was evident at the University of Brighton's Fresher's Fair, where a student group called Sex Workers' Outreach Project Sussex (SWOP) set up a stall and were handing out leaflets about the rights of sex workers, of how to get support within the immigration system and generally providing resources for support and solidarity with sex

19   www.otago.ac.nz/christchurch/otago018607.pdf.

20   www.nswp.org/sites/nswp.org/files/4.%20Impacts%20of%20Other%20 Legislation%20and%20Policy%20-%20The%20Danger%20of%20Seeing%20 the%20Swedish%20Model%20in%20a%20Vacuum%2C%20Swedish%20 Model%20Advocacy%20Toolkit%2C%20NSWP%20-%20December%202014.pdf.

workers. Not surprisingly, it was explosive. Feminist and anti-sex work campaigner, Julie Bindel, for instance said: 'This is beyond disgraceful. It makes me so angry that the sex trade's become normalised and pimped to women as though it is a harmless and respectable way to earn a living'.[21] SWOP insisted that they were not encouraging people to go into sex work, but rather responding to the fact that in the face of crippling debt, more and more students are using sex work as a way to make a living.

In the economy at large there is less job security; plummeting wages; higher unemployment; education is increasingly expensive and personal debt is rising. It's therefore unsurprising to hear that the rates of people going into sex work are also rising. 74 percent of off-street sex workers say that they do sex work because of a need to pay household expenses and support families.[22] There is also evidence showing that cuts to welfare directly cause prostitution to rise.[23] Sex work is intimately tied to the wider state of the economy and should therefore be treated as an economic, welfare and poverty issue – not as a criminal issue. As Nicki Adams from the English Collective of Prostitutes explained to me when we spoke:

> Most sex workers are mums working to support families. A lot of young people, especially working class young people, know that. They know that as a truth. They know the reality of what's going on in their own family and community much more than they want to articulate. One of the women I was speaking to recently said that when she was twelve her dad had managed to gamble all their money away. They didn't have a lot, but they

21 www.theguardian.com/education/2018/sep/30/row-over-sex-workers-support-group-prompts-university-investigation-swop-brighton-sussex (last accessed 02/2019).

22 Home Office, *Paying the Price: A Consultation Paper on Prostitution*, (2004).

23 *Star* (19 March 2014); *Star* (2 November 2016).

had enough, and he had managed to gamble it all away and from that point on and for the next 8 years she saw her mother working three jobs, worrying every week about how she was going to afford the groceries. People know that. Four million children in this country are living in poverty. Sex work is one of the ways that women have always used to make ends meet.

Chapter 12

Relationships: Just swipe right

What do we look for in a partner? In the world's very first lonely hearts posting, it was hard cash – or around £300,000 in today's money. On 19 July 1695 a London publication, *the Collection for Husbandry and Trade*, put out the following advert: 'a gentleman about 30 years of age says he has a very good estate. Willing to match himself to some good young gentlewoman that has a fortune of about £3,000 or thereabouts.' The earliest matrimonial advertisements were by and large requests for financial transactions. Perhaps the most shameless was from 1759: 'A young man wants a wife with two or three hundred pounds; or the money will do without the wife.'[1]

Today, requests for cash have been replaced by drink and dinner offers. Dating apps might be the new lonely hearts postings, but they have exploded exponentially in significance and popularity since the 1600s. In the UK, around one in four people will now meet their partner online and rates are even higher among younger generations, with almost half of 16 to 34-year-olds having used a dating app at some point.[2] In contrast, the number of

---

1 Francesca Beauman, *Shapely Ankle Preferr'd: A History of the Lonely Hearts Ad* (New York: Vintage, 2012).
2 www.bbc.co.uk/news/newsbeat-45007017.

people meeting in the traditional dating spaces, like bars, clubs and community or religious centres is falling.

Find love in a click

Tinder launched in 2012 in a world where online dating was seen by many as fringe and taboo. While controversy is never far away from anything that involves technology and sex, internet dating is now largely de-stigmatised and dominates the world of romance. It would be near impossible to list, or even find out, all the dating apps around the world today. In the UK the most popular ones range from Tinder to Grindr, Hinge, Feeld, Bumble, all the way to dating apps for people who wear glasses, beards and like vegan food. The global online dating industry is worth a whopping $4.6 billion. Match Group – the company that owned the original match.com and now has Tinder and 40 other similar businesses – pulled in revenues of $1.7 billion in 2017 alone.

Given that there are so many different dating apps catering to different people's needs, it's not easy to say exactly what it means for everyone. There are enormously popular dating apps specifically for religious people looking for marriage. SingleMuslim.com 'the world's leading Islamic Muslim Singles, Marriage and Shaadi introduction service', which had humble beginnings starting from Yorkshire, has over two million members online and has enabled over 50,000 marriages. In Germany, dating apps haven't really kicked off in the same way that they have in China, for instance, where offline dating culture is becoming more and more socially unacceptable. Tantan, the largest Chinese dating platform, has over twenty million users and claims to have created a staggering ten million couples.

Where one in five heterosexual couples meet online in the UK, a staggering 70 per cent of same sex-couples start their relationships online. In a society that assumes that heterosexuality is the norm, it's not always easy being queer and approaching someone in a bar. With homosexuality still punishable by death in five countries around the world, and the rest of the world still rife with homophobia, online platforms can provide virtual, queer-friendly spaces.

All human – and many animal – societies have had courtship rituals. But has there ever been a *true* way to date? When we look back to the history of dating, it's clear that there never was and never will be one single way of dating.

History of dating

While millennials in open or polyamorous relationships might feel like it's a new phenomenon, something that we very cleverly invented, ditching monogamy actually has a long history dating back, well, millennia. Anthropologists have estimated that only 17 per cent of human societies have ever been strictly monogamous, with the vast majority of societies embracing a mix of relationship types – with some monogamy and some polyamory, for instance. In some prehistoric nomadic communities, gathering food and resources were a constant demand and there was very rarely any extra going. Human beings and our hominid ancestors spent the past few million years or so in small, intimate groups in which adults would commonly have casual sex with multiple partners, of all genders.[3]

It is believed that farming created more fixed family models. When humans became more static, settling around urban farming centres, longterm monogamy became the norm. It's likely that at this time, there was still more space for different types of relationship, however, and as we've seen throughout the book, as nation states and other powerful religious institutions became

---

3 Christopher Ryan, *Sex at Dawn: How We Mate, Why We Stray, and What it Means for Modern Relationships* (London: HarperCollins, 2007).

the dominant model of organising society, they used violence to enforce a particular sexual morality on the people.

Monogamy was enshrined within the law and deviancy could lead to severe punishment. The very first death penalty in the whole of recorded human history was from ancient Mesopotamia and was for adultery, where unfaithful wives would be impaled on poles and displayed in the middle of the village. There were, of course, double standards – while women were not allowed to be unfaithful, men were able to have multiple wives and visit sex workers. Greek and Roman laws banned polyamony men and women were expected to live by very different moral codes. Whereas men could participate in orgies and extra-marital affairs, women would sometimes register as sex workers if they were having an affair, since adultery was only a crime that married women could commit.

There is nothing inherently philandering about men. Polyamorous societies haven't always been so stacked in male favour. In the Kingdom of Lesotho, for instance, *Motsoalle* relationships – meaning long term romantic and sexual relations between women – were not just acceptable, they were celebrated among the Basotho people. The *Motsoalle* couple would be publicly acknowledged and accepted into the community with a ritual feast, even when these women already had male partners. These practices still happen, even if they are less common now.

It was in the 1880s when dating, as we know it today, first appeared in US cities among working class communities. Dating emerged from this era due to enormous changes within the economy. Searching for work, more and more women who had grown up in small towns left their homes to find work in the cities. When they got to the cities, they would find cheap rooms, or sometimes crash with relatives. Often they might work in factories or in the homes of rich families. Some were shop assistants or secretaries. Due to more extreme conditions of poverty, African

American women were more likely than white woman to find work outside the home, mostly in domestic service. By 1900 over half of American women were working outside of the home and the vast majority of them were not married, but were dating.

Traditional parents would have preferred to set up their children through family, community or the religious institution.[4] Courting (straight) couples, however, would walk down the streets proudly holding hands. After punching out at the factory, and not having any private space of their own, they would be out in public – attending dance halls, concerts and plays together, or even just finding a dark corner to kiss in the streets. During this time, a woman's working class income was low, but having some wages did allow women to choose where they dated and with whom.

It was deeply concerning for the older generations to see young people meeting up on the streets like this. It was considered so new, so shocking and so suspicious to the authorities that they sent undercover police to spy on dating spots. One of these investigators in New York City took notes after one such surveillance mission in 1905. He wrote: The majority were 'store employees, telephone girls, stenographers, etc.' 'Their morals are loose', he wrote, 'and there is no question that they are on terms of sexual intimacy with their male companions.' In fact, in the earliest days of dating, many young women were arrested under prostitution charges. It was assumed that any young woman who would let a man take her out and buy her food and drinks could only be doing it for one reason.[5]

By the 1920s, dating had reached the US middle classes. From then until now, dating has been followed by the scent of scandal.

---

4   We're talking about heterosexual couples here, in the 1880s, homosexuality was still illegal and entirely stigmatised.

5   Moira Weigel, *Labor of Love: The Invention of Dating* (New York: Farrar, Straus and Giroux, 2017).

The eye of the beholder

Anyone who's been on the dating scene will also tell you that it's a treacherous path, lined with heartache, rejection and a lot of questionable behaviour. Previously, anecdotes would remain between friends but now the rise in dating apps has given us greater insight into people's dating lives and dating preferences. The more people that sign up to dating apps, and the more time they spend on them, the more data there is, which is good for research (and for big business).

Historically it's been thought that people tend to go for a partner who shares certain qualities with them, whether that's age, geographical closeness, attractiveness, education level or interests.

Given the uniqueness and variety of us all, you might assume it would mean we'd all have particular and individual tastes. However, dating apps have shown that our preferences are somewhat predictable. What they show may not come as a surprise. The graph opposite reveals the 'ideal' age of men and women in heterosexual dating.

Ranging from ghosting to sending explicit images, the dating world has its own moral code. Actions and attitudes that would not be acceptable in the real world are commonplace online. It ranges from men preferring younger women all the way to racial stereotyping, or sexual racism. We explored the fetishisation of people of colour and pornography, but the world of dating shows us quite how tangible the effects of racial representation are.

There was the now infamous 2014 OK Cupid survey which showed that black women were considered the 'least attractive' by straight male uses, and Asian men were also found the 'least attractive' by straight women.[6] In the US, research from Cornell University found that black men and women are ten times more

---

6 https://theblog.okcupid.com/race-and-attraction-2009-2014-107dcbb4fo6o.

A woman's age vs the age of men she's attracted to

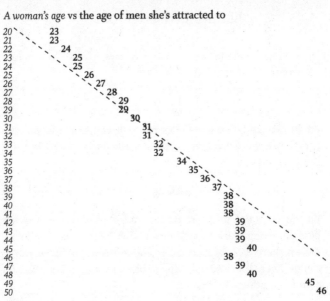

A man's age vs the age of women he's attracted to

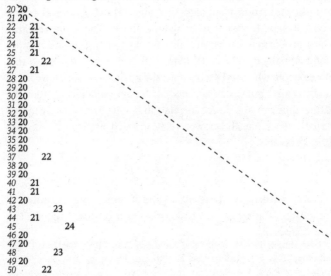

Illustration by Mona Chalabi. Source: 'Dataclysm' by Chistian Rudder.

likely to message white people than white people are to message black people.[7]

E, 20

I'm brown, and it's common for me to be called 'exotic looking' and 'fit in a weird way'. I'm constantly asked where I'm from and I'm so bored of it.

Al, 25

I'm queer and I find Grindr the easiest way to get a quick hookup. Being black though means that I come across a lot of racism there. People have called me monkey, and even worse things. I'm really tired of having to block people, or come across a profile that says 'no blacks'.

Grindr have recently launched the hashtag #KindrGrindr and an anti-discrimination campaign that aims to bring an end to the kinds of experiences that Al details above. The same research paper at Cornell University also found that using dating apps might actually creates racial bias in their users – they found that those people who used dating apps the most, were also more likely to see sexual racism as acceptable. It's no coincidence that the dating apps reveal a direct correlation between what's considered sexually desirable and power relations that exist and run deep through society.

L, 24

We all have racist parts in us, and it affects our attitudes all the time. Dating life is just another part of that. I bet a lot of

---

7   Jevan Hutson, Jessie G. Taft, Solon Barocas and Karen Levy, 'Debiasing Desire: Addressing Bias & Discrimination on Intimate Platforms,' *Proc. ACM Hum.-Comput. Interact.* 2, CSCW, Article 73 (November 2018), 18 pages. https://doi.org/10.1145/3274342.

people swipe left on someone on account of racial prejudice. We should work hard to deconstruct and try and challenge racist assumptions we have about others, in all aspects of our lives. If you think all black people are unattractive, you need to start asking yourself some pretty hard questions. But being anti-racist isn't just about these kinds of individual choices we make. To be anti-racist means being part of collective movement that directly challenges the powerful institutions upholding white supremacy. The same is said of sexism and misogyny. Undoing them will not come about from swiping right. Unfortunately it's not that easy.

Clearly dating apps are not politically neutral, and the anonymity can mean people behave terribly on them. Nonetheless, society is changing. The number of inter-ethnic marriages and relationships in the UK have soared in the last decade. In 2014, it was estimated that one in ten relationships crossed racial boundaries; and this number is on the rise. However, while the figures reflect the rising number of people of colour settling down with someone from another racial group, white people remain the most segregated – and are keeping to themselves. Nonetheless, if the trends keep going as they are, the number of mixed babies will continue to rise. What this will do for an anti-racist movement in the UK is to be seen.

Manufacturing love

Can a computer find you love? Whether you're after someone who likes hiking, or lives close to you, it's all about the algorithms. But can technology actually predict love or compatibility? In one episode of Black Mirror, it can. This dystopian society is organised through a dating system called 'Coach'. Coach collects data about the user – gathering more and more intelligence about their preferences; who they are and what makes them tick. The ultimate aim, like any good dating app, is to find 'your perfect match'. The system is so flawless that it can pinpoint, to the second, the length of time the couple will be together – sometimes it's just for the evening, for others, it's for years. But one thing is certain: the computer sets the limits to the love. In the episode, two protagonists meet each other, fall in love and their relationship is given a life expectancy that they disagree with. Ultimately, they decide to disobey the Coach and break out of the system.

Love, in the world of Black Mirror, can break all bonds. It has the power to transcend an oppressive world and release people to freedom. The Beatles sang that 'All You Need is Love', but they certainly weren't the first. Throughout history, love has been the subject of poetry, it has started wars and ended friendships.

Aristophanes, in Plato's *Symposium* put forward one suggestion. Humans were originally round: we had two faces, four arms, two sets of genitals and four legs. Legend goes, that the Gods wanted to punish humans, so Zeus cut us in half with a bolt of lighting, and from that moment, suffering entered into the human heart. According to the parable, humans wander the earth in search of our lost other half. When two halves find each other, as Plato says: 'the pair are lost in an amazement of love and friendship and intimacy, and one will not be out of the other's sight, as I may say, even for a moment: these are the people who pass their whole lives together; yet they could not explain what they desire of one another.'

This romantic ideal of soul mates carries throughout Western literature. In Charlotte Bronte's *Jane Eyre,* Mr Rochester declares his love for Jane, and echoes the belief that love in its ideal form is a physical and spiritual bond between two people:

I sometimes have a queer feeling with regard to you – especially when you are near me, as now: it is as if I had a string somewhere under my left ribs, tightly and inextricably knotted to a similar string situated in the corresponding quarter of your little frame. And if that boisterous Channel [the Irish Sea], and two hundred miles or so of land come broad between us, I am afraid that cord of communion will be snapt; and then I've a nervous notion I should take to bleeding inwardly.

There's no doubt that the dating landscape has changed since Plato and Jane Eyre's time, but does that matter? On 11 January 2013, the *New York Times* confirmed it, 'The End of Courtship?' a headline asked. The article announced that 'hang-outs' and 'hookups' had replaced the date. Philosopher Slavoj Žižek also believes that technology has taken dating and romance in the wrong direction. In his estimations, online dating is like 'drinking caffeine-free coffee', a shadow of the real thing.

But what is the real thing? Is it at Plato envisioned? Or perhaps love is gender-fluid orgies, as our neolithic ancestors believed it to be? As we've seen, the way that humans court and date has been in flux for millions of years, and today is no different. The rise of online dating reflects a changing world. And just like there was anxiety from older generations at the very advent of dating itself, today is no different. In the words of Moira Weigel who argues in *Labor of Love: The Invention of Dating*, when there's a moral panic about the end of traditional dating, it often comes hand in hand with an attempt to reinforce conservative ideals about gender and sex. Today, the young are far more tolerant and far more open about different sexual practices than any generation before us.

Conclusion

Sex education as it is taught today is outdated and ripe for transformation. In this book, I have explored other approaches and looked at new inclusive ways for young people to learn about sex and gender.

There's much more to sex than putting condoms on bananas. These pages are brimming with politics, histories and case studies in order to provide context as to *why* we are where we are. The topics I've covered, from consent to love, are intimately connected to other seemingly irreconcilable factors like capitalism, cultural and religious difference all the way to environmental degradation. Oppression and resistance have formed the way we come to understand the sexuality of others and ourselves. I have tried to forge those connections, and make clear why a sex education that does not put these political histories right at its beating heart will never succeed in empowering new generations.

That said, radical sex education on its own is not enough to challenge and fight oppression. Academic Yasmin Nair put it more plainly: 'the sad truth that many of us learn after years in sexual playing fields (literally and figuratively) is that how many people you fuck has nothing to do with the extent to which you fuck up capitalism'. The way we reproduce oppression in matters of love and lust is the necessary end result of structural inequalities that run deep throughout our world. To challenge them will extend far beyond reading this book.

This book is aimed at a group of people who are considered beyond the age where sex education is needed. It's true that – hopefully – you should have been taught about puberty, menstruation and the basics of how to practice safer sex, but what about a more developed, nuanced and critical understanding of sex? Human relationships are complicated and messy, they are subject to change, euphoric one moment, violent and life-changingly destructive the next. If #MeToo taught us anything, it's that sex education must be lifelong.

Resources

Mental Health Support

Youth Access: Support, advice and information about counselling in the UK for young people.

Nightline: Provides confidential and anonymous emotional support to students in distress.

Campaign Against Living Miserably (CALM): Support for young men aged 15 to 35 suffering from depression.

Eating Disorder Support

Anorexia and Bulimia Care: Provides advice and support to anyone affected by an eating problem.

Men Get Eating Disorders Too: Information and advice for men on eating disorders.

Sex and Gender

TranzWiki: Directory of all groups campaigning for, supporting or assisting trans and gender non-conforming people in the UK.

Gendered Intelligence: Support and campaigning group for young trans people 18 to 24.

Mermaids: Support group for young trans and gender non-conforming people.

The UK Intersex Association: Support for intersex people and campaigning group for intersex people's rights.

Contraception and Abortion Advice

Brook: Brook provides free and confidential sexual health services and advice for young people under 25.

Marie Stopes: Reproductive and sexual health services and support, specifically abortion support and care.

Consent and Sexual Violence

NUS I Heart Consent Campaign: Education campaign about consent in universities and colleges across the UK.

NHS support: Find your local rape and sexual assault support centre: www.nhs.uk/Service-Search/Rape-and-sexual-assault-referral-centres/LocationSearch/364.

Rape Crisis national freephone helpline: National freephone helpline on 0808 802 9999 (12–2.30 p.m. and 7–9.30 p.m. every day of the year).

IMKAAN: The only UK-based, second-tier women's organisation dedicated to addressing violence against Black and minority women and girls.

Broken Rainbow: Support group for LGBTQ+ people who have experienced sexual or domestic violence.

Muslim Women's Helpline: Support group for Muslim women who are subjected to sexual or domestic violence.

Sexuality

Stonewall: Major charity within the UK that works to achieve equality and justice for LGBTQ+ people.

LGBT Switchboard: LGBT+ helpline for support, advice and information.

IMMAN: Support group and charity for LGBT Muslim people, their families and friends.

Sex Work

English Collective of Prostitutes: Network of sex workers campaigning for decriminalisation and safety.

Sex and Relationships

Sexpression: Student-led charity that empowers young people to make decisions about sex and relationships.